Bharata Natyam on the Global Stage

At Home in the World

PERFORMING ARTS SERIES

General Editor :
FARLEY P. RICHMOND

Vol. X

Bharata Natyam on the Global Stage
At Home in the World

<u>*Other Vols. in the Series :*</u>

I. **Indian Theatre:** Traditions of Performance
—*Farley P. Richmond, Darius L. Swann* and *C. Shapiro* and *Phillip B. Zarrilli*

II. **Sanskrit Drama in Performance**
—Eds. *Rachel Van M. Baumer* and *James R. Brandon*

III. **Sitar Music in Calcutta:** An Ethnomusicological Study
—*James Sadler Hamilton*

IV. **Drama and Ritual of Early Hinduism**
—*Natalia Lidova*

V. **Sanskrit Play Production in Ancient India**
—*Tarla Mehta*

VI. **Sitar Technique in Nibaddha Forms**
—*Stephen Slawek*

VII. **Sitar and Sarod in the 18th and 19th Centuries**
—*Allyn Miner*

VIII. **The Dictionary of Hindustani Classical Music**
—*Bimalakanta Roychaudhuri*

IX. **Semiosis in Hindustani Music**
—*José Luiz Martinez*

Bharata Natyam on the Global Stage

At Home in the World

JANET O' SHEA

MOTILAL BANARSIDASS PUBLISHERS
PRIVATE LIMITED • DELHI

First Indian Edition : Delhi, 2009
Earlier Published by Wesleyan University Press
Middletown, Connecticut

ISBN : 978-81-208-3362-3

MOTILAL BANARSIDASS
41 U.A. Bungalow Road, Jawahar Nagar, Delhi 110 007
8 Mahalaxmi Chamber, 22 Bhulabhai Desai Road, Mumbai 400 026
203 Royapettah High Road, Mylapore, Chennai 600 004
236, 9th Main III Block, Jayanagar, Bangalore 560 011
Sanas Plaza, 1302 Baji Rao Road, Pune 411 002
8 Camac Street, Kolkata 700 017
Ashok Rajpath, Patna 800 004
Chowk, Varanasi 221 001

Designed and typeset by Juli Allred, BW&A Books, Inc.

PRINTED IN INDIA
By Jainendra Prakash Jain at Shri Jainendra Press,
A-45, Naraina, Phase-I, New Delhi 110 028
and Published by Narendra Prakash Jain for
Motilal Banarsidass Publishers Private Limited,
Bungalow Road, Delhi 110 007

Contents

Illustrations

Acknowledgments

This book is based on seventeen years' experience with bharata natyam. More people extended support to this project than I can acknowledge here. I thank, first, Nandini Ramaṇi and Susan Foster, who have been with this project since its beginnings in 1989 and whose generosity, critical guidance, and tutelage have shaped my thinking and my dancing.

I also want to thank those who read drafts of this text, who commented on public presentations based on this material, and who have offered support both intellectual and emotional. Specifically I thank Jens Giersdorf, Indira Viswanathan Peterson, Tim Shireman, and Lakshmi Subramanian for specific feedback and encouragement. Thanks to Ananya Chatterjea, Emilyn Claid, and Davesh Soneji for critical and supportive comments on the ideas in this text. I would like express my gratitude to Parama Roy and Piya Chatterjee, who commented on earlier versions of this material and who helped bring it into its current form. Thanks also to Kay Poursine for introducing me to bharata natyam. The memory of Cynthia Jean Cohen Bull runs through this text; in bringing both kindness and intellectual rigor to the earliest work I did on this subject, she impelled me forward.

I extend gratitude to the dancers who took the time to discuss their work with me. In particular, Mayuri Boonham and Subathra Subramaniam of Angika, Shobaṇa Jeyasingh, Mavin Khoo, Hari Krishnan, Lata Paḍa, Menaka Thakkar, Usha Srinivasan, Lakshmi Viswanathan, and Chitra Visweswaran gave freely of their time and their thoughts. Here, too, I would like to acknowledge Nandini Ramani and her daughter Sushama Ranganathan for offering me a home in Chennai and for introducing me to that city's dance milieu. Jeyanthy Siva was kind enough not only to provide me with introductions in Toronto but also to offer me a place to stay in Jaffna. Vinodhini Sachidananda and S. Ravindran provided translation and research assistance in Jaffna and in South India, respectively.

This research benefited from funding from a diverse range of sources. Most recently, the Association for Asian Studies provided a subvention grant for the publication of this text. The Arts and Humanities Research Council enabled the completion of the manuscript by awarding me a Small Grant in the Creative and

Performing Arts and by funding the AHRC Research Centre for Cross-Cultural Music and Dance Performance, of which I was part. I conducted research in India in 1999 through the University of California, Riverside Graduate Dean's Doctoral Dissertation Research Grant and in 1995–96 under the auspices of the American Institute of Indian Studies Senior Performing Artist Fellowship. A UC Riverside Humanities Predoctoral Fellowship, 1996–2001, provided support for this work, as did funding from UC Berkeley for completion of my master of arts degree in South Asian studies.

Finally, I would like to thank the editorial board and staff of Wesleyan University Press and BW&A Books, Inc. In particular, I thank Suzanna Tamminen, Leslie Starr, Barbara Norton, and Julie Allred for the care and attention they gave to this project.

Preface

In August 2001, the dance critic and historian N. Pattabhi Raman published an article entitled "What Is Bharata Natyam?" in the South Indian dance and music periodical *Sruti*. In this essay, he raised questions over the quality, classicism, and integrity of the dance form and suggested parameters for its maintenance. He argued that some innovations to bharata natyam's structure and vocabulary diluted the classical practice, while others retained its values but kept it up to date. He therefore called for sub-fields within bharata natyam in order to differentiate between classical dance and the contemporary genres that draw from it. As part of this argument, Raman urged the formation of an experts committee and of an accompanying "blue book" that would establish a code for what lay within the limits of the classical form and what lay beyond.

This publication happened to coincide exactly with the completion and public release of my Ph.D. dissertation. There, I argued that twentieth-century bharata natyam consisted of a set of contrasting, sometimes competing, opinions, viewpoints, and choreographic visions. I posited that both diversity and contention characterized the form, rendering it impossible to fix or pin down. My first reaction, therefore, to Raman's article was apprehension. Here was a critic whose work I respected greatly and whose writing, in some important arenas, underpinned my own. Yet he had urged for classification, for the reestablishment of boundaries, while I suggested that bharata natyam set the pace and that critical frames adjust to the practice and allow the dance to move forward.

Revisiting Raman's concerns has raised some important insights for me and therefore helped to shape this book. Most apparently, Raman's argument indicates the importance of boundaries: classical forms and their practitioners value and, in some cases, demand parameters. Classicism promotes rigor and integrity and, therefore, according to one persuasive line of reasoning, it requires standards, not just of quality but also of identity; a classical practice cannot include everything and still be classical. People train in and view classical dance genres for different reasons than they pursue contemporary or popular forms, and one of these reasons has to do with clarity.

However, that the need has arisen to outline bharata natyam's parameters explicitly suggests that Raman and I were pointing to the same phenomenon: that the current moment constitutes a crucial juncture in bharata natyam's history. Dancers, critics, and viewers debate its form, content, structure, and identity. The dance practice, depending on one's opinion, is flourishing or fracturing, burgeoning or fragmenting. But there is little doubt that it is changing.

In this text, then, I want to account for the complexity of this moment as well as for the intricacies of bharata natyam's equally complicated twentieth-century history. I still maintain that this dance practice incorporates diversity and divergence. As I shall argue, dancers from the 1930s to the present have come up with remarkably different understandings of bharata natyam's identity and history, let alone how to perform allegiance to them. It is this tendency within the form—that of finding different solutions to the same question—that I want not only to foreground but also to support. For these reasons, I am inclined to accept change as part of this dance form's history.

This doesn't mean, however, that I propose that dancers and viewers celebrate all modifications as equally beneficial. I want debates over quality, rigor, and the politics of representation to continue. I would like to see dancers, choreographers, and dance writers ask, as Raman did, for example, whether bharata natyam is a movement vocabulary or a set of compositions, considering whether ensemble pieces contribute to the bharata natyam repertoire or only pieces that are part of the traditional solo *margam* qualify. I think we should keep asking these questions; I just don't think we should necessarily lock down the answers to them.

As a result, I do not seek to provide a single answer to any of the questions I raise in this text. This book does not evaluate the merits of particular investigations or praise some choices at the expense of others. Rather, the pages that follow draw out the content of these different projects, highlighting what claims practitioners make, through reference to what arguments, and how these contentions line up with the concerns of their historical context, that is, with their social, temporal, and political environments. What appears in the body of the text is therefore less a linear argument than a genealogy of the multiple meanings that a particular dance form can have.

The central tenet of my argument remains that this space of exchange, debate, and argument defines the form. I want this text to account for the diversity of the bharata natyam field, because I believe this vitality characterizes some of the best aspects of the dance form. I strive here to continue a tendency toward debate in the bharata natyam sphere, encouraging critical thinking about choreographic practice. In this text, I raise issues—those concerned with contrasting choreographic choices, their politics of representation, and the strategies of self-definition that accompany them—that, I hope, will spark further discussion among performers, choreographers, critics, viewers, and scholars. I foreground the complex politics of representation embedded in choreographic practice so that practitioners can make more conscious choices as to where they wish to position their work. One question, then, that I want to continue asking pertains to the social, political, and cultural implications of redefinitions of form. Since 1989 I have seen bharata natyam dancers critically extract and reflect upon the principles and strategies of its past practice. It is this tendency, and not just diversity alone, that I wish to support. I believe that this approach, more than adherence to specific aspects of classical practice in itself, will foster a form that continually engages and challenges its viewers

Most important, I want to see bharata natyam thrive, preferably as more than a museum piece or a respectable avocation. The solo format contains a clear aesthetic logic and a remarkable rigor; it challenges the audience by layering meaning and rhythm and by weaving different interpretations together in the interplay between gesture, song, and movement. Although some artists have retained this tradition of complex understatement, others have drifted into confectionery entertainment. In some cases, the elements of the dance practice that I value most—a powerful yet calm demeanor, a strong female stage presence, and an active relationship between dance and music—have diminished in the interest of soliciting audience approval. Certainly one way of resisting a move toward commercialization is through recourse to tradition. But it doesn't always follow that a solo dancer offers a more meticulous presentation while ensemble choreography is lighter and simpler. Allegiance to classicism is not the only device for countering negative changes to a practice. Experimental solutions provide equally interesting challenges; some such inquiries appear in this book.

Bharata natyam is a resolutely global form. It has circulated internationally at least since 1838. In the last two decades, however, this circulation has accelerated; its viewers, too, are on the move. A dancer can no longer assume that she performs for an audience of aficionados. Dancers need to find new, critical, and reflective solutions to ongoing dilemmas, whether those occur in the devising of dances themselves, in their theatrical presentation, or in the discourse that surrounds them. Changing audience points of view, shifts in funding structures and objectives, and a surplus of dancers mean that choreography needs to adapt in order to continue. It also will need to change—and has changed—to garner the attention of international audiences. The question here, too, is not whether bharata natyam will transform, but how. I am not suggesting that choreography should be simplified in order to accommodate a global viewing public; rather, performers can adapt, and have adapted, strategically, acknowledging multiple viewerships while continuing to stimulate considered reception. A look to the past may be helpful, not to reconstruct the form or fix the values of an older practice but to examine the strategies deployed by earlier performers in order to make more conscious decisions about what to change, why, and how.

Bharata natyam is not in danger of dying out. The question is not whether bharata natyam continues or not; its continued existence is, I believe, a given. But this certainty doesn't guarantee a secure future. My concern is how the dance will develop and in which directions. Will it become more and more of a sideline, a training in heritage and culture, for girls and young women who discontinue dance after marriage or who embark on other careers? Will it continue its forays, resolutely and unapologetically, into the so-called dance mainstream of the global stage? Or will it remain relegated to the "world dance" or "community" margins? Will it challenge its audiences, in India and abroad, attracting new viewers while providing familiar spectators with material to ponder?

I think that performers, choreographers, and viewers can address these concerns by reflecting on bharata natyam's recent past. I would like to see bharata natyam dancers and viewers acknowledge what the form has already achieved by grappling with the concerns of a globalized modernity and the political concerns of local, regional, and national identities, and use these accomplishments to look forward. I also hope that dancers, viewers, and critics will look at the tactics of the past and consider extracting—or reformulating—these strategies in order to apply them to new situations. In fact, I believe that bharata natyam will survive best as a dynamic, contemporary form if it has this kind of a future.

Rather than requiring a new set of parameters, I think that bharata natyam dancers deserve credit for opening up arenas of debate, dialogue, and difference within a "traditional" form. Other forms that define themselves as classical grapple with similar dilemmas: performance styles that identify themselves as traditional do so through reference to boundaries as well as to past practice. Likewise, dance traditions that characterize themselves—or are characterized by others—as "national" or as regionally specific include some elements of practice and avoid others so that choreographic decisions dovetail with particular politics of representation. The issues raised here, then, also appear in other dance practices, including, for example, ballet, the "national" dance genres of West Africa, and some articulations of modern dance. Bharata natyam dancers, by meeting the challenges that confront them, not only address issues in their own sphere but also provide solutions useful to practitioners of other forms. Bharata natyam led, albeit problematically, the recontextualizing of traditional forms in India in the early to mid-twentieth century. Perhaps it can now be at the forefront of a different movement: the incorporation of "traditional," "ethnic," and "national" forms into the mainstream of an international dance milieu, assuring that a range of dance forms does not just appear on but also questions the assumptions of the global stage.

Introduction: Performing Politics in an Age of Globalization

Stage lights come up gradually to the sound of a *tambura*'s drone. A dancer clad in a colorful tailored sari and adorned with jewelry emerges from the wings. To the accompaniment of a flutist's leisurely melodic exploration, she walks calmly, but deliberately, to center stage. The sinuous melody concludes, and a staccato phrase begins as the dancer's feet articulate a sharp rhythm. Signaled by the *nattuvanar*'s, or musical conductor's, crisp syllables, the dancer launches into a virtuoso phrase of abstract movement. Her legs rotate out from their parallel position as she simultaneously strikes the floor with her foot and sinks her weight into a deep, bent-legged position. Hands and fingers curve into precise shapes that ornament the attacks of her footwork. Her still torso floats over her dynamic feet. She rotates to reach forward while her weight stays firmly grounded. She concludes by briskly repeating this final movement as her feet strike out a pattern over which her torso and arms arch.

The virtuoso phrase, identified in classical aesthetic terms as *nritta*, rhythmic abstract or nonthematic dance, ends as suddenly as it began. The dancer walks backward, feet and legs hemmed in to a parallel position, the vibrancy of the pulsative choreography retained in her clear enunciation of each step. As she steps forward again, the tone of both the music and the dance changes. Her feet move through a walking pattern that, although simple, illustrates the *tala*, or rhythmic structure, of the accompanying song. A vocalist sings lyrics that the other accompanists follow as the music becomes fluid and melodious. The dancer has launched an *abhinaya*, or dramatic dance, section. Her movements are leisurely yet focused. Expressive hands trace their way through the space in front of her body as she looks at them with careful attention, lifting her gaze to the audience to emphasize a point and turning her attention to places on the stage to invoke other characters. She augments her hand gestures with facial expressions so that a dramatic scenario unfolds: she is elated, but her joy is so excessive that it overwhelms her; she is worried and penitent, then angry and frustrated. A line of sung poetic text repeats as she develops variations on this theme.

This dancer performs a *varnam*, an item of classical bharata natyam reper-

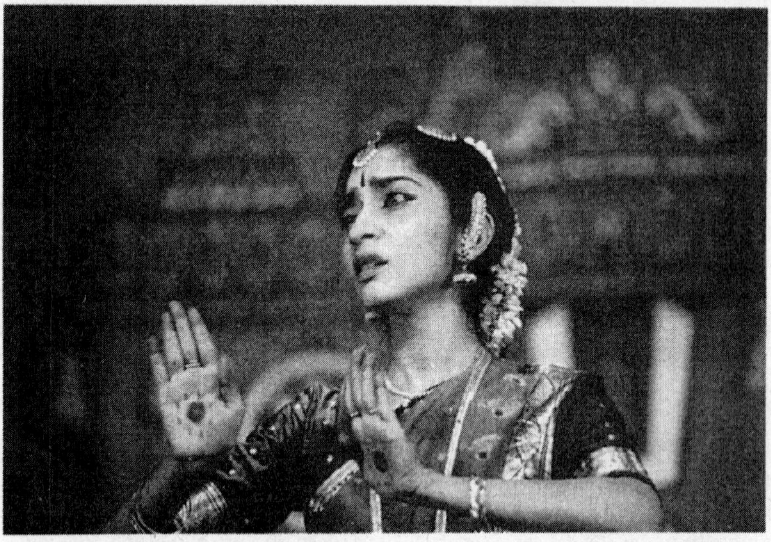

Figure 1: Sushama Ranganathan performing a varnam. Photograph by author.

toire characterized by such juxtapositions between nritta and abhinaya or *nritya*, expressive choreography. The dance, with its clarity and precision, distinctive vocabulary, and identifiable syntax, seems pristinely classical. The dancer, too, looks unshakably traditional in her vibrant costume, in the jewelry that ornaments her head, face, neck, and arms, and in the ankle bells that grace every movement with added sound. She may be a young South Indian woman dancing on a stage in a Chennai theater where women in silk saris and men in neat starched dhotis watch attentively as ceiling fans whir overhead. Then again, this dancer may be performing in a community center in Manchester, a temple in San Jose, or a major venue in New York, Toronto, or Mexico City. The dancer may be not a young South Indian but rather a second-generation Bangladeshi Briton or a French, Japanese, or Argentine performer. The dancer may be not a sari-clad South Asian woman but rather a man from Singapore or Australia.

At the beginning of the twenty-first century, the global status of bharata natyam renders the form ever more visible. For instance, London's Greenwich Dance Agency's autumn 2002 series featured, as part of the citywide Dance Umbrella festival, contemporary classical works by Vena Ramphal, Mavin Khoo, and Angika's Mayuri Boonham and Subathra Subramaniam, as well as Shobana Jeyasingh's modernist choreography based on the bharata natyam movement vocabulary. During the 1990s and in the first decade of the twenty-first century, the Canadian choreographers Lata Pada, Hari Krishnan, Menaka Thakkar, and Sudha Thakkar Khandwani staged new work at Toronto's prominent Harbourfront

Centre. Mythili Kumar's bharata natyam company performed at San Francisco's Fort Mason. Chandralekha, a contemporary choreographer at the forefront of the Indian modern dance movement who, like Jeyasingh, uses bharata natyam as a primary source for the creation of new work, presented *Raga* at the Brooklyn Academy of Music. No longer relegated to the so-called world-dance margins of a global performance milieu, bharata natyam appears alongside European and North American forms in mainstream venues.

Nonetheless, the form continues to suggest exotic allure, with bharata natyam performers adorning the covers of guidebooks and travel brochures, their beauty luring tourists to India—as if such images didn't also appear at local theaters in Chicago and Stockholm. Classical Indian dancers framed Madonna's performance for the 1998 MTV Music Video Awards, the troupe offering the performance an aura of exotic distance that the singer's access to a group of local Los Angeles dancers belied. Dancers, promoters, and critics describe the dance form as homogenous and esoteric, applying terms such as "ancient" and "traditional," not informing audiences that even classical dancers create original works, often outside the conventional solo concert format.

The dance form, and especially its amateur practice, also provides a means for immigrants to maintain their social identity in diaspora. It offers South Asian communities in Europe and North America an implement for, in Arjun Appadurai's (1996) terms, intentional cultural reproduction and, thus, for the reiteration of their homeland's culture in diaspora. Parents encourage their daughters to study bharata natyam in the hopes of their performing an *arangetram*, or solo debut. The arangetram, for many young women, marks their entry into a middle-class diasporic Indian community rather than into the performance milieu, often terminating a period of dance study instead of inaugurating a dance career.[1] Although a renowned choreographer may present her version of bharata natyam in a prominent venue and in a choreographic form that lines bharata natyam up with Western contemporary dance and ballet, the performance of Indian heritage attracts many of her students and, more particularly, their parents to her dance classes.

Bharata natyam in North America has seen decades of training in diaspora, beginning in the 1970s when bharata natyam schools sprung up alongside the influx of upper-middle-class immigrants with science and technical degrees who relocated to the United States and Canada to work in computing and engineering fields (Srinivasan 2003). These immigrants were mainly men, and they brought with them wives and daughters who drew on their educational and artistic backgrounds and founded dance schools. Although South Asian dance has had a longer history in the United Kingdom, there, too, it experienced both a surge and a streamlining in the 1970s, with the foundation of the arts organization Akademi and the decision to align classical Indian dance with the British independent dance sector. Although performers trained in diaspora may have been encouraged to study dance by parents or relatives interested in acculturation, they have used their dance study to produce choreographies unexpected by earlier generations. It is likely that this impulse will continue, so that parents send daughters to bharata natyam classes for immersion in Indian culture and heritage, as well as to acquire aesthetic accomplishments. Some of these same daughters will then use bharata natyam to query their own position interrogating the expectations both of immigrant communities and of the European and North American dance mainstream.

Bharata Natyam, Globalization, and the Politics of Revival

Bharata natyam transcends national and cultural boundaries yet remains resolutely tied to them. It circulates globally but operates as a symbol of the exotic. Performers put forth contrasting versions of the dance form in performance, even while some still describe it as part of a fixed, unbroken tradition. Dancers and promoters present the practice as high art and performers struggle to ensure that Western contemporary dance forms make room for it on the global stage. It offers a means of identity production for diasporic communities, who then take the opportunity it provides to refigure the dance form and to query their social, cultural, and political situations.

How to account for such a complex situation? I suggest that explanations for these apparent contradictions lie in the form's twentieth-century history and, more specifically, in the period from 1923 to 1948, known as the bharata natyam revival.[2] Performers, critics, and promoters brought bharata natyam to the urban proscenium stage, recontextualizing and renaming it. In doing so, they crafted a genealogy in which bharata natyam came to represent ancient tradition and critical experimentation, nationalism, regional identities, and the global transference of forms outside of geographical and cultural boundaries. In the 1920s through the 1940s, the form's continuation depended on its relationship to politics. During this period, dancers contended with political imperatives that altered the practice and the context in which it occurred. They addressed these concerns by crafting choreographic interpretations that offered varied positions on the debates of their time.

Bharata natyam's immediate predecessor was *sadir*, a primarily solo dance form practiced by *devadasis*, courtesans affiliated with temples and courts as performers and ritual officiants. The anti-nautch (literally, "anti-dance") reform movement, begun in 1892, denounced the devadasis' nondomestic lifestyles as prostitution and their ritual activities as superstition, while also criticizing the ostensible lasciviousness of the dance they performed. The colonial assumption of direct rule in southern India and the resulting demise of the patronage system, as Avanthi Meduri (1996) and Hari Krishnan (2004) indicate, also prompted the disintegration of the devadasi system and the practice of sadir. The anti-nautch reform agitations, together with changed political circumstances and economic conditions, impelled the form into obscurity.

In 1927, a group of activists and arts supporters formed the Madras Music Academy after they organized a music conference to accompany the first South Indian meeting of the anticolonial Indian National Congress. In 1931, the tide turned for dance as the academy's officers took interest in sadir and included a performance by devadasis in its concert series. A better-attended concert followed in 1933 (Arudra 1986–87a; Gaston 1996: 288–311). By 1935, the form had begun to change hands, with middle-class, Brahman girls and women, such as Kalanidhi Narayaṇan, Lakshmi Sastri, and Rukmini Devi, turning to dance study and performance and thus enhancing the respectability of bharata natyam. The new dancers, together with critics and venue organizers, defended the formerly marginal practice by aligning it with political discourses such as nationalism and regionalism. This intersection of dance with politics worked in two ways: political concerns validated bharata natyam while the classical features of the dance form substantiated claims to political legitimacy. Bharata natyam thus moved from the edges of South Indian cultural life to the center of its most intense social and political contentions, including those over national independence, regional identity, and caste and class status.

Nonetheless, the transformation of a disreputable practice into an emblem of cultural identity remained incomplete. Performers, in response, validated the form and justified their decision to practice it through arguments that circumvented or reclaimed the devadasi legacy. The revival of bharata natyam therefore depended not only on politics, but also on the ability of practitioners and promoters to articulate their understanding of the dance form's history.

By 1933 the Music Academy's members had renamed sadir; it was now bharata natyam, an appellation that associates the form with the canonical Sanskrit aesthetic theory text, the *Natyasastra*, and its author, Bharata. It is also described as an anagram of *bhava* (mood or emotion), *raga* (melody), and *tala* (rhythm), and is erroneously, if popularly, mistranslated as "Indian dance-drama." All of these associations served to validate the dance by shifting its points of reference from a marginalized local practice toward ancient, pan-Indian traditions such as Sanskrit drama and aesthetic theory and by invoking the aesthetic categories that support India's two classical music systems: Hindustani and Carnatic music. The revival's dancers and promoters presented concerts, lectures, and demonstrations and built up a body of critical and scholarly writing on bharata natyam that addressed its formal qualities, history, and cultural significance. These histories, in turn, paralleled and supported efforts to imagine communities (to use Benedict Anderson's [1991] term) consisting not only of the nation but also of the region and the urban center.

The transformations that bharata natyam underwent in the revival also placed it within a global dance milieu. The forced transnationalism of colonialism had

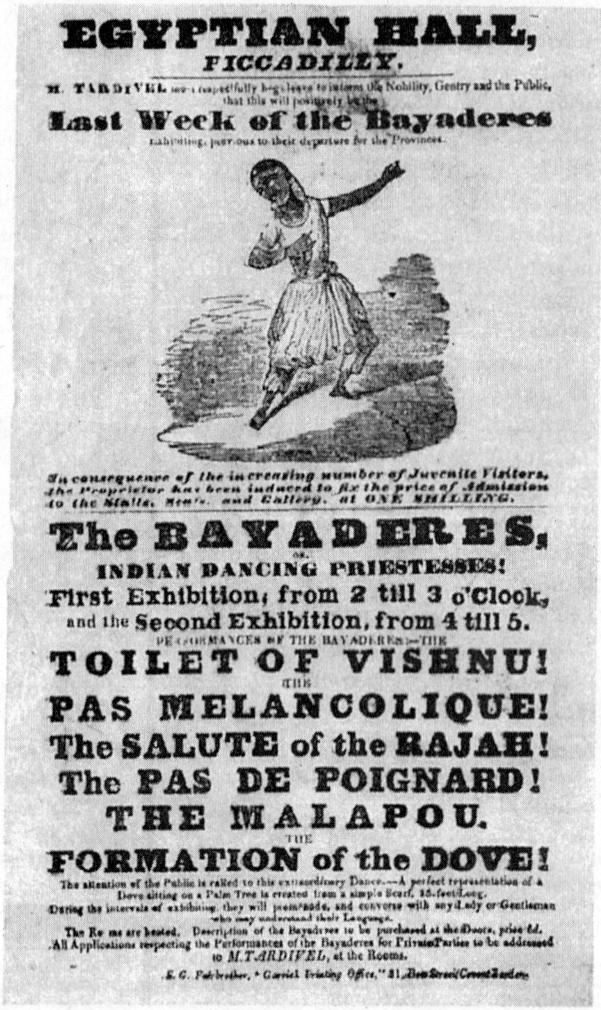

Figure 2: Advertisement for a performance by the devadasis of Pondicherry, Egyptian Hall, London, 1838. © V & A Images/ Victoria and Albert Museum.

introduced European, universalist, post-Enlightenment values to Indian social life, which, in turn, prompted the reform of Indian cultural traditions and social practices. Dance and the institutions that supported it did not escape this overhaul of Indian cultural life. Rather, the performers who reconfigured bharata natyam in the 1930s engaged with the concerns of the colonial social reform movements of the nineteenth century and with the modernization of Carnatic music, a process that had begun in the eighteenth century but accelerated in the nineteenth and twentieth centuries (Allen 1998; Subramanian 2006).

Bharata natyam also entered the urban concert stage following a long period of Western fascination with "the East" and with India in particular. This preoccupation found its expression in dance practice when, for instance, European promoters sponsored performances by the devadasis of Pondicherry in London and Paris in 1838. In the late nineteenth century, European and North American choreographers offered their own interpretations of "Eastern" themes through, for example, the Orientalist ballet *La bayadère*, which claimed to depict the life of an Indian temple dancer, a tradition that premodernist interpretive dancers such as Ruth St. Denis then brought forward into the twentieth century.

This Orientalist fascination focused not only on India generally but also on its dance forms. This interest subsequently fueled the bharata natyam revival. St. Denis performed *Nautch Dances* in India in 1926 and raised the interest of her urban, middle-class audiences as to the nature of the dances that inspired her interpretations (Allen 1997; Coorlawala 1992). The American dancer Ragini Devi, born Esther Sherman, began her career as a St. Denis–style "oriental" dancer but relocated to India in 1930 in order to train in classical Indian forms; she spent the following years performing and lecturing on the merits of India's traditional dances and participated in the Music Academy's 1933 conference. The ballerina and choreographer Anna Pavlova created a series of "Oriental"-themed dances and subsequently traveled to India to find the dances on which her sketches were based. She was disappointed to find the solo female forms virtually nonexistent but discovered a means of rectifying the situation when she met Rukmini Devi, a South Indian Brahman theosophist. Pavlova's suggestion to Rukmini Devi to find her own dance form initiated a historic move when the latter returned to India and sought out devadasi dance. Pavlova had earlier influenced the Indian modern dance forerunner Uday Shankar, who, at the time, was studying art in London. Shankar's collaborations with Pavlova prompted his entry into choreography and dance performance in Europe and India. He embarked upon a project that not only sent him to Europe and North America but also drew him back to India, where he helped spark the career of the revival-era devadasi dancer Tanjore Balasaraswati. Balasaraswati subsequently enjoyed a global reputation, finding admirers among international audiences that included premodern and modern dancers such as Ted Shawn and Martha Graham.[3]

Although European and North American modernists used the images they created of the "mystical East" to demonstrate their own singularity (Chatterjea 2004a; Srinivasan 2003), their strategies paralleled those of the bharata natyam revival. Premodern and early-modern dancers alongside ballet revivalists such as Pavlova reclaimed dance that was maligned in Europe, as in India, as idle entertainment associated with prostitution. Bharata natyam dancers, like Western dance modernists, strove to validate dance, describing it as a "high," autonomous art that expressed creativity and engaged with serious intellectual and philosophical concerns. Dancers in India, as in the West, validated their performance practice by emphasizing the originality of their work while also drawing on historical sources for their inquiries.

The revival installed bharata natyam as an independent concert dance form; it

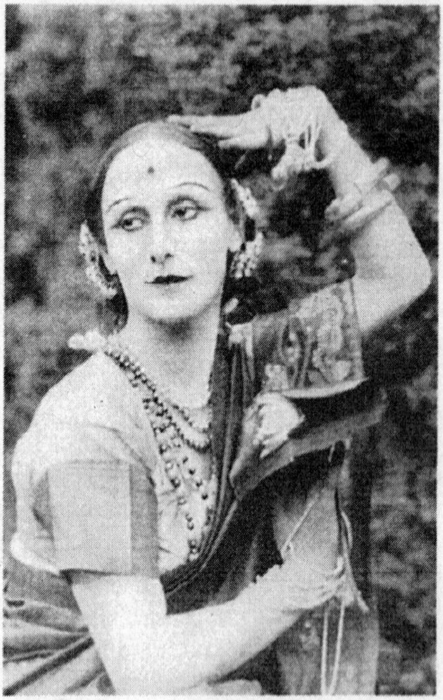

Figure 3: Anna Pavlova's *Hindoo Dance,* 1923. Program from a performance at the Royal Opera House, London. Photograph by E. O. Hoppè. © 2006 Curatorial Assistance, Inc., Los Angeles. Photograph Courtesy of V&A Images/Victoria and Albert Museum.

positioned the dance practice not as a ritual activity associated with temples and courts but as an urban, global art, crosscut by concerns of local, regional, and national identities. The legacy of this period, which established bharata natyam as what it is today, extended into subsequent decades. The era's complexities, investments, and contradictions inflected twentieth-century bharata natyam so that later interpretations of the form emerged out of the transformations initiated during the revival. In the pages that follow, I suggest that dancers continued to contend with concerns of historicity, national identity, regionalism, gendered respectability, locality, and the transnational circulation of dance practice while also reflecting on them differently from their early-twentieth-century counterparts. Engagement with new historical and social contexts shifted debate in new directions, which encouraged choreographic positions on these issues to both fragment and multiply.

Twentieth-century bharata natyam, then, articulated the concerns of a complex history in which political debates played themselves out on a choreographic field. Key social and political issues faced by urban, middle-class Indians and diasporic South Asians in the twentieth century expressed themselves in this performance practice. Not only did large-scale discourses inflect bharata natyam, but performers, in making decisions about composition, form, and the represen-

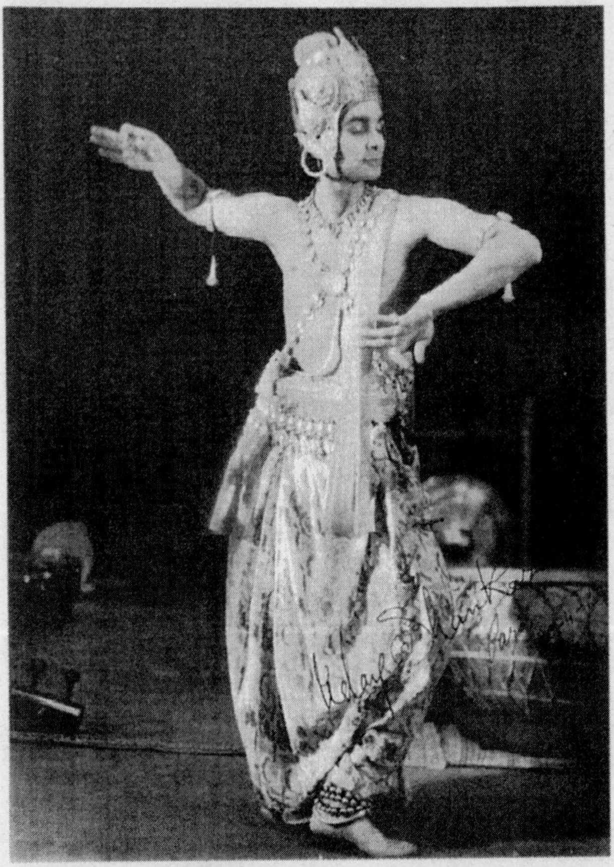

Figure 4: Uday Shankar. Courtesy of Jerome Robbins Dance Division, The New York Public Library for the Performing Arts, Astor, Lenox and Tilden Foundations.

tation of the dance practice, also raised political questions alongside aesthetic ones. Such concerns overlaid dance practice but did not dictate it. This web of social contentions both informed twentieth-century bharata natyam and enabled its practitioners to represent their own views on the form and on the politics that surround it.

Choreography, Politics, and Agency

This is, therefore, a book about the global cultural politics of the twentieth century as expressed through choreography. Dancers and viewers, especially in Europe and North America, do not usually think of dance as playing a role in political life. For many, dance is either a pleasant diversion or an unfettered expression of creativity. Dance scholars have argued in response that dance, far from being an autonomous and fringe venture, speaks directly to the social and political concerns of its temporal and cultural context.

In this study, I rely upon the insights of writers who examine the political investments of movement practices.[4] I also draw on studies particular to bharata natyam that are positioned within South Asian studies and that use anthropology, ethnography, ethnomusicology, postcolonial theory, and performance studies. These inquiries address the bharata natyam revival as a product of Indian colonial history, locating in the dance form the tactics of anticolonial nationalism.[5] Moreover, I deploy a body of literature from postcolonial studies that investigates the consolidation of Indian national identity through "cultural"—that is, not overtly political—devices such as literature, music, film, television, domestic and ritual practice, education, and language.[6] I bring together these three approaches in order to formulate the central arguments of this study. First, I suggest that the recontextualization of bharata natyam from the 1920s to the 1940s developed in response to, but was not wholly restricted by, the nationalist movements of the late nineteenth and early twentieth centuries. I then go on to argue that bharata natyam practitioners aligned their projects with political discourses through an explicit and selective engagement with the dance form's past; divergent interpretations of form, history, and identity express themselves in choreography. Finally, I maintain that bharata natyam's intersection with political discourses at "home" and its encounters with international dance milieus enabled practitioners to cultivate new local identities in a global context.

This book, although it builds on sociological, anthropological, performance-studies, and postcolonial-theory projects that illustrate the relationship of bharata natyam to politics, also represents a departure. Unlike earlier studies, this text locates these strategies in particular dance examples. Using choreography as a metaphor for the decisions made not only in composition and creation but also in discursive representations of the dance, in teaching, and in performance, I examine how practitioners carved out their positions on history, tradition, nationalism, regionalism, gender, and local identity in the work they did onstage and in dance classes as well as in their commentaries on the form. In the pages that follow, I argue not only that political agendas have affected bharata natyam, but also that the practice of dance provides a performer with strategies for grappling with social and political concerns. I therefore use the term choreography to invoke the conscious process of selecting some movement material over others, whether for use in performance or instruction.[7]

The definition of choreography is a source of debate in Indian dance criticism and scholarship. For example, the *kathak* innovator Maya Rao argues that only work that significantly challenges the form or the content of conventional classical or folk dances should be identified as choreography (2001: 82). She advises dancers not to "confuse choreography with arrangement or re-arrangement of dances" but to apply the term to original creative ventures (83). The Canadian bharata natyam practitioner Menaka Thakkar, by contrast, maintains that her creation of new pieces with novel structures developed out of an evolutionary process from performance to instruction to composition. Because an instructor incurs responsibility for repertoire, including the compilation of phrases, Thakkar suggests that teaching gives a dancer the opportunity to create movement sequences as part of the transmission of conventional items of repertoire. Thakkar sees a continuum between the assembling of conventional items of repertoire and the crafting of evening-length ensemble pieces (personal correspondence 1998, 1999).

The influential postmodern choreographer Chandralekha defines choreography as "the science of organizing movement in space" (2001: 66). In the essay in which she offers this definition, Chandralekha urges dance practitioners to give measured attention to the structures and devices of choreography in order to produce more rigorous dance compositions. Chandralekha focuses on means for developing the quality of and care given to new projects in the Indian dance sphere. However, the definition she provides is broad enough that it can be applied to work that its composer defines either as experimental or as classical.[8]

Given these contrasting definitions of "choreography," I use the word to recognize a range of practices, extending its definition beyond the experiments of a self-defined innovator to include a number of activities in the dance class, rehearsal studio, and onstage. In using the term broadly, I do not suggest that every dancer is automatically a choreographer. Rather, I restrict the appellation choreography to situations of explicit decision making about performance, training, and presentation. I recognize the need to distinguish among contemporary and "traditional" projects and the desire on the part of many innovative practitioners for audiences to acknowledge that they push the boundaries of their forms, but I do not think the term choreography is the best device for making this kind of identification. I would suggest, rather, a delineation between classical, modern, and postmodern aesthetics. Part of this process involves untangling what Ananya Chatterjea calls the "masking of the choreographic process" in the Indian classical dance sphere (2004a: xi).

As I use the term here, then, choreography includes the arrangement of inherited works and decisions made in improvised performance as well as the composition of original pieces by a self-defined innovator. Likewise, it includes the reconstruction of movement based on textual description or visual imagery. In deploying this term, I do not restrict choreography to its most common usage: the invention of a movement vocabulary or the creation of a new work in its entirety. Rather, the notion of choreography here incorporates decisions about structure, content, and performance context. In the case of bharata natyam, these choices frequently run alongside a discursive articulation of histories for the dance practice and allow a performer to address the concerns of a social, cultural, and political context. In making decisions about performance and how to represent the dance form, dancers stake out their own positions within the debates that surround the practice. As such, choreography—decisions made about dance performance and training—provides a means of negotiating a complex of discourses.

This book, then, is also about agency. Locating individual agency in a practice may seem to echo the celebration of the autonomous subject of previous decades and centuries. The poststructuralist critique, and particularly the Foucauldian concern with discourse as social and bodily inscription, represented the independent subject as a humanist fantasy. Those working with performance used this idea to unravel the romantic and modernist notion of the inspired genius, untouched by social surroundings. Such arguments gave scholars a way of looking at artistic practices as elements of social life that engage with broader concerns. This critique broadened study from the form itself to its intersection with a larger context.[9]

At the same time, however, an emphasis solely on the subject-position as a site of political inscription returns us unwittingly to an old-fashioned notion of dance (and other artistic practices) as "reflecting" its social environment. In looking at the South Asian context, a deconstruction of personal decision making can run close to an Orientalist notion of individuals replicating tradition, with practitioners constrained by, rather than actively negotiating, their heritage. Traditional scholarship has tended to render hereditary practices outside the West as fixed, denying the authority of non-Western artists in their own fields while foregrounding the self-sufficiency of their European and North American counterparts. In such a situation, a wholehearted anti-humanism replicates the Orientalist assumption of a static, unselfconscious culture that simply reiterates itself through its practitioners. For this reason, although critical, and especially poststructuralist, history contested the idea of individuality, postcolonial theory, anthropology, and sociology have foregrounded personal agency (Appadurai 1996; Blacking 1981; Chatterjee 1993; Inden 1990; Visweswaran 1994).[10]

My discussion of choreography represents an attempt to intertwine two perspectives. I suggest that practitioners select from a range of possible options and, in doing so, creatively respond to larger social and political discourses. I identify choreographic practice as tactic and strategy, focusing on action and decision making.[11] The metaphor of strategy rather than, for instance, that of creation acknowledges that broader concerns—social, political, cultural, and economic—inform a dance tradition. Unlike the image of inscription, however, strategy suggests that although broader issues shape choreographic practice, they do not determine it (Foster 1995: 3–21; Novack 1990: 141). I thus attempt to highlight an interplay of social, political, and aesthetic concerns, while recognizing that dancers grapple with these issues in a range of different ways and through devices and decisions that are not easily or obviously predictable from their social identity, their stylistic lineage, or their performance history. Such an approach recognizes that the political pressures of a particular cultural and historical moment constrain the choices an individual makes. Yet it also acknowledges the tactical nature of those decisions.[12]

Twentieth-century bharata natyam dancers inherited a legacy of colonial reform, a nationalist imperative to represent cultural identity through reference to the past, and a globalization of dance innovation. Performers grappled with nationalist and regionalist ideologies, contended with a conflation of women with tradition in their representation of the form, and relied upon transnational discourses on dance. They did not, however, simply reiterate the claims made by political activists, by venue organizers, or by Western dance modernists. Rather, in developing choreographic strategies, they carved out subject positions that allowed them to represent their own understanding of bharata natyam's identity and its past, as well as of gender, class, national, regional, and local affiliations.

In looking at the twentieth-century history of bharata natyam, I do not aim to recover an independent dancer-subject. Politically interested individuals drove the effort to bring bharata natyam to cosmopolitan urban centers, and, thus, the present-day form is anything but autonomous. For these individuals, promoting and modifying a dance form was, in itself, a political act that would bolster nationalist feeling. Bharata natyam dancers thus positioned their choreographic practice on the concert stage through its ability to accommodate broader concerns. However, interpretations of the form diverged as soon as bharata natyam's introduction to politics began. The politics of representation embedded in these decisions varied accordingly, and, thus, dancers have come up with remarkably different, creative iterations of social investments.

Political agendas frame choreographic choices, but practitioners deploy these discourses to their own ends, coming up with results that the initiators of political movements may not expect. In crafting choreographic representations, dancers claim an agency that has the potential to disrupt, as well as to contribute to, the dominant forces of their immediate context. This process is one of resistance as well as capitulation, contestation as well as consensus. Dancers participate in a local production of meaning that, I argue, remains central to twentieth-century bharata natyam despite its numerous transformations and displacements.

I see this book as part of an argument for understanding the global through the specific. Dance works articulate politics of representation and speak to the immediate local contexts in which a globalized form appears. Divergent interpretations of bharata natyam circulate globally, but they produce meanings that are profoundly local. This text places the local into discussions about transnationalism.

Choreographing History in Colonial and Postcolonial Politics

Critics, dancers, and scholars who have queried the recontextualization of bharata natyam in the early twentieth century have seen it as a transformation as well as a restoration. Yet some performers, promoters, and viewers, both within and outside the form, still label bharata natyam as unproblematically, consistently traditional, classical, and ancient, fixed and untroubled by modern concerns. In such portrayals, bharata natyam's identity is self-evident. Those defending tradition and those pitting themselves against it frequently treat tradition as a fixed and singular entity.

This book, by contrast, represents an attempt to understand bharata natyam not by looking to history for sanction, but by examining historiography as a device that dancers use to develop their own interpretations of their dance practice. I suggest that tradition is not a static source from which present-day choreography flows but is, instead, a way of viewing the past that varies from one dancer to the next. My emphasis on competing understandings of bharata natyam comes out of a desire to query narratives that treat the dance form as homogenous and static. It is also an attempt to account for the divergent versions of the dance form's past and present state that I have seen appear onstage, in dance classes, and in discussions about the form.

The attention I give to multiple understandings of tradition and classicism stems from my training in bharata natyam. I entered this field in 1988 as a student of the Thanjavur court style of bharata natyam associated with the legendary dancer T. Balasaraswati. I began studying bharata natyam as an undergraduate at Wesleyan University with Balasaraswati's student Kay Poursine and traveled to India in 1989 to study with Balasaraswati's senior disciple, Nandini Ramani. My connection to Balasaraswati was indirect: she had died in 1984, four years before I began studying bharata natyam. My tutelage occurred under her students.

Coming to bharata natyam from outside of India and the South Asian diaspora raised a particular set of questions and placed my inquiry in a specific situation, the elements of which frame this text. I trained in bharata natyam in Connecticut and in California as well as in Madras (now Chennai) and performed it not only in India and the United States, but also in other countries, such as Mexico, the United Kingdom, and the Philippines. This experience, I suggest, is not anomalous. Rather, it exemplifies the global positioning of bharata natyam. My own practice of the form, therefore, pushed me from the outset to account for the transnational circulation of Indian classical dance forms.

In addition, learning bharata natyam not as a child in India or in an Indian community setting but as a university student in North America facilitated my access to Balasaraswati's dance style and, hence, to her understanding of history. Despite the renown that Balasaraswati enjoyed as a performer, her style remains marginal to the bharata natyam milieu. Instruction in Balasaraswati's style is rare and located almost as much in North American universities as in the private arts venues and schools of Chennai. Nandini Ramani and her daughter Sushama Ranganathan teach in Chennai, and Balasaraswati's daughter Lakshmi Shanmukhan Knight returned frequently to Chennai while living and teaching in New Jersey until her death in 2001. Among the hundreds of bharata natyam schools and teachers in Chennai, only these three belong to Balasaraswati's stylistic lineage. Likewise, although a few private institutions in North America are dedicated to the propagation of Balasaraswati's style, such as Lotus Music and Dance (New York), the Balasaraswati School of Music and Dance (New Jersey), the Center for World Music (California), and Priyamvada Sankar's school (Montreal), Balasaraswati and her disciples tended to find sustained support in university contexts: Balasaraswati taught at Wesleyan University, as did her daughter Lakshmi and her disciple Kay Poursine. Balasaraswati also held residencies at Mills College and California Institute of the Arts. Another of Balasaraswati's students, Meda Yodh, taught at the University of California, Los Angeles. Thus, my entry into the bharata natyam field in a North America university brought me to a style that would otherwise have been hard to find; at the same time, it occurred in circumstances that immediately encouraged me to contextualize the information I was given.

Training in bharata natyam involved immersion in history. However, I encountered a different understanding of history, through the Balasaraswati legacy, than I would have if I had trained in an Indian community setting. Other dance writers, notably Avanthi Meduri (1988) and Vena Ramphal (2003), speak of an oft-recounted narrative that accompanies training in bharata natyam technique. In this account, bharata natyam fell into decline and was rescued by the pioneers of the 1930s. Through my study of Balasaraswati's style, I encountered an alternate understanding of the revival. The history I first learned of the form was one of disappearance and disintegration. For Balasaraswati, bharata natyam was a South Indian tradition that found its proponents in the hereditary community of devadasis. She traced an unbroken chain from the artistic practices of the eighteenth- and nineteenth-century Tamil courts to twentieth-century bharata natyam. Attempts in the present to alter, improve, purify, or modernize bharata natyam, she maintained, would sever this connection. A profound sense of loss accompanied this version of history. I found Balasaraswati's iconic figure compelling and the history of bharata natyam that she had described convincing. This image of a living yet marginal legacy threatened by its very popularity drew my attention as much as the technical complexities of the form did. Nonetheless, I struggled with the idea that the form required preservation and resisted change, that its standards of excellence could only be found in its past and not in its future.

During my first trip to India in 1989, I encountered the interpretation of bharata natyam that Meduri and Ramphal speak of. Research led me from back issues of *Sruti* magazine to the Sampradaya archive, where I found other periodicals such as the *Kalakshetra Quarterly*.[13] Here, dancers put forth another understanding of the past: the new generation of practitioners, exemplified by Rukmini Devi, rescued a dance form that had reached its nadir, reelevating it to the status it had enjoyed in ancient times. In this account, the devadasi tradition that Balasaraswati valorized symbolized, or at least coexisted with, this deterioration. Rukmini Devi and her students located the authenticating past of bharata natyam not in the nineteenth-century Thanjavur court, but in ancient traditions such as Sanskrit drama. For Rukmini Devi, the twentieth century was a time of rejuvenation, not of threatened destruction.

Through this inquiry, it emerged that history—ever present and taken for granted—also constituted an arena of debate. History was, therefore, selective: practitioners such as Balasaraswati and Rukmini Devi presented their understandings of it by emphasizing some aspects of the past and eschewing others. From 1989 to 1994, although I focused on building a performing career in the United States, I continued to grapple with the question of a multiply defined past. I undertook a master of arts in South Asian studies and investigated Indian colonial politics and postcolonial theory. Through critiques such as those leveled by Hayden White and the Subaltern Studies Group, I came to view history as the choice of some elements of the past over others and therefore as both a construct and a symptom of modern concerns and conflicts.

Such insights informed my attempts to outline the differences I saw between Rukmini Devi and Balasaraswati: their interpretations of history articulated different politics of representation. Rukmini Devi's agenda aligned clearly with that of cultural nationalism in that she positioned bharata natyam as an emblem of indigenous self-respect through which India's distinctive cultural attributes and its ancient traditions became manifest. Balasaraswati's performance and pedagogical practice intersected less explicitly with large-scale politics, but her emphasis on the Tamil tradition and on South Indian literature and music shared strategies with regionalists of Tamil Nadu. Each practitioner also took a different stance on the gender politics of colonial India. Rukmini Devi located, in dance, a place of power and authority for the middle-class, upper-caste woman who would improve the tradition, while Balasaraswati defended a marginal caste and class through a celebration of the devadasi legacy. Their identities and agendas seemed to line up into sets of opposing categories: Rukmini Devi privileged a Sanskrit tradition, Balasaraswati a Tamil one. Devi identified bharata natyam as a national form; for Balasaraswati, its roots were specific to southern India. Devi celebrated the new generation of Brahman (upper-caste) practitioners, while Balasaraswati maintained that the form rightfully belonged with the lower-caste devadasi practitioners who had nurtured it for centuries. Devi saw herself as purifying and revitalizing a form in decline, while Balasaraswati strove to uphold a threatened tradition. Rukmini Devi and Balasaraswati, then, frequently staked out contrasting positions on key debates surrounding the form.

Thus, my early research, which began with an article I wrote in 1994 and published in 1998, explored different definitions of tradition in bharata natyam. This constituted my first foray into the divergence of meaning and form that I had witnessed in the bharata natyam sphere. I attended to the inquiries of these two practitioners, investigating both their similarities and their differences as emblematic of the discourses of the revival. The fundamental tenet of this work—that revival-era bharata natyam incorporated a range of interpretations of history, tradition, and classicism as well as of social and political identities—informs this text. Nonetheless, subsequent developments, both in the dance field and in my thinking about it, challenged this binary representation of definitions of history.

When I returned to India in 1995, I encountered a dance scene in which new works, and new understandings of bharata natyam's identity, form, and history proliferated. Although I realize now in retrospect that this process began in the mid- to late 1980s, with, for example, Chandralekha staging her groundbreaking *Angika* in 1985 and Padmini Chettur presenting her first contemporary experiment in 1989, the 1980s simultaneously saw a boom in classical dance training and performance. Classicism dominated the Madras dance scene in the late 1980s, an aspect that informed my view of bharata natyam in 1989.

In 1995, by contrast, new choreographic ventures seemed ubiquitous. What I found particularly striking, though, was that many of these ventures demonstrated historical ties. That is, I rarely saw new works that engaged in experimentation for its own sake without locating its inquiry through reference to history. And yet, the versions of history that I encountered departed from the binary oppositions I saw in the work of Rukmini Devi and Balasaraswati. Rather, particular components of performance and different aspects of history could be taken apart and refigured in a range of ways. Lakshmi Viswanathan's staging of *Vata Vriksha* (*Banyan Tree*), on January 1, 1996, brought this point home for me. The piece has a Sanskrit title, and its choreographer is a middle-class Brahman woman who followed in the footsteps of Rukmini Devi, receiving her training as a result of the events of the revival. Nonetheless, Viswanathan identified *Vata Vriksha*, in an onstage introduction, as "the story of the dance of [her] people," that is, Tamils. Like Balasaraswati, Viswanathan foregrounds the early devadasi legacy, draws from Tamil poetry, and highlights the accomplishments of the Thanjavur courts. Yet, like Rukmini Devi, she treats the nineteenth century as a period of decline and distances her vision of bharata natyam from the remaining twentieth-century devadasi practice. The piece concludes with a celebration of the efforts of Devi and of the revival.

This work provided a history that, to me, was surprising. Viswanathan references sources similar to those Balasaraswati used by invoking the Tamil literary canon. She foregrounds the temple and court dance traditions but, like Rukmini Devi, celebrates a distant past, albeit a Tamil, not pan-Indian one. As did Devi, she represents the mid-twentieth century as a time of restoration, not of threatened disintegration. Here, definitions of history no longer split into the sets of oppositions I had identified in the work of Rukmini Devi and Balasaraswati. A choreographer could celebrate the revival, in general, and Rukmini Devi, in particular, while tracing a Tamil history for the dance, drawing together the divergent sources that Balasaraswati and Devi appealed to. Upon encountering this and other equally complex narratives, I realized that I could no longer fix bharata natyam even as a site of contestation or of divergence. Rather, I noted that although history and politics continued to run through discussions about bharata natyam, there were as many configurations of such associations as there were dancers.

Nonetheless, I still see the positions of Rukmini Devi and Balasaraswati as fundamental to a discussion of the bharata natyam revival. Both figures held sway over the bharata natyam milieu throughout the twentieth century. Although their instructional lineages are not necessarily the most prominent in the bharata natyam field today, the perspectives that the two artists brought to bear endured, especially because each created a series of commentaries on their own work through articles, talks, and presentations as well as through their pedagogical and performance endeavors. Each established a discursive position, through the remarks they produced, through instruction, and through a body of repertoire, that continued to influence decisions made in the late twentieth century and into the present.

For these reasons, I treat each dancer as paradigmatic of an approach to a particular issue. It is precisely these differences and the ways in which the dancers realized their contrasting perspectives that laid the conceptual and choreographic groundwork for the revival. Because my aim here is less to understand their differences in themselves and more to account for the impact of their complex legacies on the bharata natyam field, I argue not for the discreteness of their projects, but rather for their positions as two poles of a dialectic, out of which twentieth-century bharata natyam emerges as its synthesis.[14] I draw out these perspectives, suggesting a dialogic relationship and a complementary opposition between the two. Each chapter begins with an investigation of the divergent views that Rukmini Devi and Balasaraswati held. I complicate this dichotomy by locating similarities in their projects, identifying points where their work met and where they retained elements of the other practitioner's argument. Indeed, that their work met at key junctures enabled the very contrast I have described.

My aim is not to propose an evaluative comparison between the two artists, to rank them hierarchically, to measure the contribution of each to the bharata natyam field, or to determine who was more successful, influential, or aesthetically "better."[15] Instead, I explore the strategies mobilized by each practitioner, including their approaches to training and performance, their different understandings of bharata natyam's past, and the tactics they used to legitimize the dance form. I then argue that their divergent points of view, as well as the principles upon which they agreed, not only drove the revival but also laid the ground for twentieth-century bharata natyam. Their divergent discursive perspectives contributed to the repertoire of choices that dancers draw from today.

Each of the sections that follows sets up a fundamental concern of the bharata natyam revival and tracks the articulation of this issue in the different aesthetic and political positions taken by Rukmini Devi and Balasaraswati. For example, as I shall argue in chapter 1, both practitioners described their work as traditional, yet they handled training, performance, and composition in contrasting ways. This indicates that they defined tradition, and indeed history, differently. Nonetheless, both dancers agreed on the importance of historical practice: they concurred that the dance form should adhere to its origins in order to retain its most important aesthetic values, even as they diverged in how they understood this past.

However, these two figures were not alone in initiating the bharata natyam revival. I therefore examine the influence of other contemporaneous figures on the revival, indicating the intersections and disparities in their perspectives. I likewise attend to the investments of the institutions, such as the Madras Music Academy, Kalakshetra, and Tamil Isai Sangam, that supported these dancers, acknowledging that the perspectives of the individual performers sometimes diverged from those of the organizations through which they presented their work. This study thereby extends my earlier investigations, considering choreographic endeavors that include the cross-gender performances of the revivalist and dancer-impresario E. Krishna Iyer, the transnational dance projects of Ragini Devi, a North American interpretive dancer who turned to classical performance, and the experiments of the early modernist Uday Shankar. I frame these viewpoints less as a set of discrete epistemologies and more as a configuration of options, the components of which dancers continue to refer to and reflect upon today.

Both when I entered the bharata natyam field in the late 1980s and as I continued my dance study in the 1990s, I encountered diversity in choreographic practice and in definitions of tradition and classicism. At the same time, writers, dancers, and promoters continued to refer to the bharata natyam revival; publications such as *Sruti* and *Kalakshetra Quarterly* made frequent mention of this period. That the revival was important even at a time of divergence prompted me to consider how the concerns of this period articulated themselves in the late twentieth century. Dancers in the 1990s still seemed to feel the need to legitimize their practice of the form, indicating that bharata natyam, at least in some quarters, retained associations with its marginal past. Practitioners and critics debated parameters for change, and performers put forth divergent understandings of what comprised classical aesthetics. I found that late-twentieth-century work also embodied affiliations with national and regional identity, contentions over gendered respectability, and local identities. As a result, in this book I carry the distinctions that revival-era practitioners deployed forward into the late twentieth century and suggest that these perspectives provided models for subsequent generations of practitioners to develop their choreographic choices.

I argue here that the revival and the late twentieth century accommodated two different generations of performers, not that they formed discrete eras. Balasaraswati and Rukmini Devi lived and worked until the mid-1980s, so their careers overlapped with those of late-twentieth-century dancers, a number of whom received their training in the 1940s, 1950s, and 1960s. Nonetheless, the key contentions of the former diverged from those of the younger generation as each group framed its decisions in response to a different set of social, political, and economic concerns. In other words, new contexts required contrasting strategies from those of the revival. The chapters that follow also address the changing social and political circumstances of the late twentieth century. New situations combined with the enduring importance of the revival encouraged dancers to engage with and reconsider the tasks undertaken by performers such as Rukmini Devi, Balasaraswati, and E. Krishna Iyer. Late-twentieth-century dancers reflected critically upon the strategies of the past, creatively rearranging and reinterpreting the approaches deployed in the revival as they enabled them to contend with the social and political concerns of a global dance milieu.

The Body of the Text: Structure, Titles, and Reading Strategies

I define bharata natyam broadly in this study, including choreography beyond that of the conventional solo concert format or margam. I attend to projects whose initiators stand outside the classical milieu because I want to investigate contestation as well as consensus over bharata natyam's identity. The parameters of a practice define it as much as its center does. Moreover, what is at the margins now may become conventional in the future. Yet this book does not only examine the work of those who push the boundaries of the form. It also concerns itself with those who establish them and who identify themselves as classical practitioners.

This text does not provide a comprehensive account of twentieth-century bharata natyam or even of the bharata natyam revival. It would be difficult to do justice to all the dancers who added to the development of the twentieth-century form; others, such as Sunil Kothari (1979) and Anne-Marie Gaston (1996), have tracked the key contributions of major performers in detail. I am more interested here in contending with issues—the aesthetic, social, and political concerns that emerged in the course of bharata natyam's recontextualization and that remained central to the twentieth-century history of the dance form—and in invoking specific dance examples that engage with these points of discussion. I have relied, in this process, on those whose work enjoyed critical attention which, therefore, provided me with substantial documentation. (Attending to the forgotten figures of bharata natyam would have been a separate project in its own right.) Likewise, although some luminary dancers and choreographers appear only briefly, while others feature more prominently, their inclusion in this text is not intended as a hierarchical indicator of quality. Rather, I have focused on examples that intersect, in interesting and striking ways, with the issues I see as arising in the form.

In this text, I sketch out, in Foucauldian terms, an archaeology, not a history. I do not trace a linear history of twentieth-century performance, but rather look at two time periods—the revival and the late twentieth century—that I see as pivotal to bharata natyam's recent past and present: the first years saw the dance form's recontextualization, while the latter witnessed an upsurge of its popularity and of choreographic production. Each, for different reasons, prompted a corresponding, rhizomatic growth of contrasting interpretations of bharata natyam's history, identity, and form.

In order to accommodate two time periods as well as varied interpretations of form and history, this book mobilizes a series of intersecting dialogues, each of which highlights one area key to twentieth-century bharata natyam: tradition and individuality, nationalism and regionalism, reform and revival, and urbanization and global circulation. These tensions are dialectical, not dichotomous. Although at first glance opposing pulls may seem to foster the development of two camps of bharata natyam dancers, I argue that these contrasting positions provide a repertoire of options that performers configure in different ways. They proffer a set of possibilities from which individual dancers derive their own interpretations of bharata natyam. Twentieth-century bharata natyam emerges as the synthesis of divergent tendencies.

The structure of the varnam undergirds the design of the chapters of this text. Rather than tracking the causal development of events in time, a varnam evinces a single dramatic moment, layering it with images, references, and a range of meanings and allowing one interpretation to lead into the next. This trajectory leads into a fresh take on the initial subject. In these chapters, too, one perspective does not yield, by the force of narrative flow, into another. Although they contend with two separate eras, the sections that follow investigate different issues that arise in the same moment and similar concerns that appear across historical periods but are reflected on in contrasting ways. This study does not follow a linear path toward a singular conclusion, nor does it trace a chronological journey from one representation of bharata natyam into subsequent versions of the form. Rather, it explores the same issues at contrasting times, opening them up into further inquiries, deepening and broadening the discussion of particular concerns. Conversely, from one chapter to the next, I investigate a range of issues in similar historical moments, approaching dance work and promotional projects from alternative angles and deriving new interpretations from this changing view.

Each chapter adheres to a similar structure: I introduce an area of debate, track its emergence in and through Indian colonial politics, reflect on its articulation in the revival and in the late twentieth century, and consider a critical interrogation of this issue by a choreographer who works with the movement vocabulary of bharata natyam but outside the classical sphere. All four chapters open with commonplace assertions about bharata natyam: that the dance form is "traditional" and, hence, ancient, for instance, or that it is essentially feminine. The chapter then goes on to challenge that observation through reference to the historical circumstances that gave rise to its emergence, tracing a genealogy of that assumption. In the process, I introduce two competing concerns, such as tradition and innovation, and follow their articulation in their late-twentieth-century form back to events that preceded the bharata natyam revival. The second section of each chapter thus draws out an area of debate within Indian colonial politics as it affected the development of particular imperatives in the bharata natyam milieu. Similarly, the third section of each chapter frames the changed perspectives of the more recent social context as they affect the sets of imperatives in question, before moving on to outline how several late-twentieth-century dancers contended with these issues. The bulk of each chapter attends to the consideration of the matter in question through dance examples as well as through promotional, scholarly, and pedagogical practices in the revival and the late twentieth century. All chapters conclude with an investigation of a choreographer who works against the issue with which classical practitioners grapple and who therefore provides a different angle from which to reflect upon these concerns. In short, the first two sections illustrate the focus of the chapter, identifying a key issue and establishing its stakes, and the latter three sections root the debates—and challenge them—through specific choreographic examples.

Chapter 1, "Tradition and the Individual Dancer," investigates tensions between continuity and individuality in twentieth-century bharata natyam. I examine the social and political factors—such as the impact of colonial Orientalism, nationalism, and the global circulation of dancers and choreography—that encouraged the explicit discussion of continuity and creativity in dance praxis. I argue that performers responded to colonial criticism as raised in the anti-nautch movement to abolish dance in Hindu temples and as expressed through the Orientalist valuation of ancient texts and traditions. Bharata natyam practitioners put forth different definitions of history that validated contrasting aspects of the dance form and, in doing so, supported their own understandings of creativity. As a result, tradition and individuality did not necessarily work at odds. Rather, contrasting ideas of continuity lent themselves to particular understandings of creativity and vice versa.

Chapter 2, "Nation and Region," suggests that the interpretations of history proposed in the revival intersected with the production of imagined communities. The bharata natyam revival, as I shall indicate, hinged upon the dance's intersection with nationalism. However, bharata natyam was not simply reformulated in the interest of the nation-state. Rather, it emerged as a space where different communities could be imagined and cultivated. Dancers defined the nation in contrasting terms while also positing diverse understandings of the dance form's relationship to the region and its languages. The chapter identifies the influence of divergent strains of nationalism and regionalism in the contrasting approaches of specific practitioners while also suggesting that politics manifested in different ways in the dance milieu than it did in public arenas concerned with language and governmental politics.

The title of chapter 3, "Women's Questions," is a play on the nineteenth-century phrase "The Woman Question," which referred to the concerns raised about the status of women in society by the protectionist-reformist and early feminist movements, in both colonies and metropoles. In this chapter, I argue that although twentieth-century bharata natyam dancers negotiated colonial, European feminist, and nationalist perspectives on the status of women, they also used such debates as vehicles for crafting their own identities within the dance milieu and in the public sphere more generally. In this chapter, following Amrit Srinivasan (1983, 1985), I argue that bharata natyam dancers of the early twentieth century grappled with the reformist and revivalist discourses that had brought the "Woman Question" to center stage at same time that campaigners had pushed dance to the margins of public life. Likewise, using Partha Chatterjee's (1993) theorization of the nationalist categories of "home" and "the world," I suggest that the nationalist consolidation of femininity undergirded the refiguration of bharata natyam. However, I maintain here that the issues raised in this refiguration endured not only because dancers were subject to ideals of womanly respectability, but also because they deployed them to craft their own positions in the dance sphere, and, thus, these categories remained highly productive for subject formation.

Finally, chapter 4, "The Production of Locality," draws its title from Arjun Appadurai's (1996) argument that globalization has produced novel kinds of social affiliation that root themselves in new physical or virtual spaces. In this chapter, I argue that revival-era practitioners struggled to validate a form that had been not only marginalized but also displaced; they strove to integrate bharata natyam into the hybrid city of Madras while also positioning it in relation to a globalized dance milieu. Drawing on Matthew Allen's (1998) and Lakshmi Subramanian's (2006) work on music and Indira Viswanathan Peterson's (1998) study of Tamil literature and theater, I examine the expression of local affiliation in dance as it helped to establish Madras as an urban arts center. Through this process dancers developed localizing strategies that incorporated colonial and indigenous hybridities. In establishing bharata natyam as capable of consolidating new, urban identities, practitioners crafted a form that could accommodate difference. Such strategies, in turn, allowed them to negotiate the concerns of a global dance arena. Performers carried these approaches forward into the late twentieth century, enabling bharata natyam to affiliate itself with more distant environments, such as the metropolitan centers of Europe and North America.

It is this accelerated global circulation and its accompanying relocalizing that have given *At Home in the World* its title. I want to call attention to bharata natyam's initial displacements, first from its sites of performance in temples and courts, then from its new homes in the cities of India. At the same time, I suggest that through the South Asian diaspora, performers' global career trajectories, and international interest in Indian classical dance, bharata natyam dancers relocalized the form. In doing so, they crafted a response to (neo-)colonialism, economic globalization, and the marginalization of non-Western forms by international arts spheres. By relocalizing the form, they gave it the ability to accommodate new belongings. A look at the thriving bharata natyam scenes in cities outside India, such as London, Toronto, and the greater San Francisco and Los Angeles areas, corroborates this impression.

The title of the book also comes out of the theorization, addressed in chapter 3, of the gendering of cultural identity in colonial and postcolonial India. The bharata natyam revival hinged on a nationalist "remaking of Indian women" (Roy 1998) while also departing from it. Bharata natyam practitioners, over the course of the twentieth century, have used gender debates to cross the perceived boundary between the "feminine" home and the "masculine" world. The global circulation of bharata natyam illustrates this process: women who initially appeared as emblems of authentic cultural tradition became its ambassadors internationally. Bharata natyam's complex twentieth-century history, when viewed closely, splits apart a gendered binarization of spheres. This intricacy and hybridity renders bharata natyam neither a derivativ reaction nor a static cultural artifact, but a dynamic method of engagement with a changing world.

The breadth of methodologies and subject matters examined here has encouraged me to write this text with multiple audiences in mind. I have therefore elected to include more information—especially on South Indian colonial and postcolonial politics—rather than less. Because an understanding of Indian political history is crucial to appreciating the divergent directions that bharata natyam has taken, the chapters incorporate a discussion of major political issues as they pertain to the dance debates in question. Some readers may find this material familiar; it may be new for others. I thus suggest a range of reading strategies: those well acquainted with Indian history and politics may want to skim the second sections of chapters, which outline overarching political issues, before focusing in on the articulation of these concerns in contrasting approaches to bharata natyam. Readers who are less familiar with colonial politics may wish to consult the appendices, which explain, in greater detail, the cultural and historical background of these movements. Likewise, for readers less accustomed to the vocabulary used to describe Indian classical dance forms, I have provided definitions of key terms in the text and included them in a glossary.

In keeping with the varnam metaphor, this book ends where it began: with a discussion of bharata natyam's past in relation to its future. Like the aesthetic inquiry of the varnam, however, this process is not merely circular. Instead, the text returns to the initial question with alternate points of view in mind, with new issues raised and different interpretations suggested. Through these discussions, it emerges that bharata natyam stands, on the one hand, in relation to social and political issues endemic to the Indian social landscape of the twentieth century. On the other hand, these concerns travel across the world's stages. The dance practice developed into a contemporary, urban, concert art informed by the investments of the nation, the region, and the urban center and expressed through notions of gendered reputability. This complex history has created a series of double binds in which dancers, instructors, writers, and viewers expect bharata natyam to be verifiably traditional yet creative, authentically Indian yet globally accessible, respectable yet commercially viable. The very pressures that inflect the form, however, also provide the opportunity for dancers to represent their own perspectives in choreographic practice. This, in turn, allows for the self-fashioning of the dancer's identity as she addresses a global dance milieu. Bharata natyam is therefore both haunted and enabled by its own contentious history. Its past will continue to inform its present. The question for viewers and performers is how these influences will occur and what aspects of the past will carry forward. At present, perhaps more than at other moments in time, practitioners, writers, and spectators can use the past to frame new questions that will, in turn, push bharata natyam in unforeseen directions.

1: Tradition and the Individual Dancer

History and Innovation in a Classical Form

Critical accounts and promotional materials frequently refer to bharata natyam as "ancient." The dance form's status as traditional and classical seems to render it fixed, even timeless. A connection to the past appears to be a given for this dance practice. Even on closer examination, a relationship to the past seems integral to the dance form's identity, its content, and its structure. Present-day bharata natyam choreography draws from the dance practices of earlier decades and centuries. Its movement vocabulary derives from sadir, the solo dance performed by temple and court dancers in precolonial and colonial South India. The margam—the concert order that determines when in a program each dance piece appears—was standardized in the nineteenth century by the renowned musician-composers of the Thanjavur Quartet. The roots of bharata natyam extend still further back. For example, the *mudras*, or hand gestures, used today accord in both shape and meaning with those described in the *Natyasastra*, a Sanskrit dramaturgical text, dating from the beginning of the Christian era. Similarly, an arangetram, or initial performance, described in the fifth-century Tamil epic *Silappadikaram* correlates with that of devadasi practitioners of the nineteenth century, which then established the protocol for twentieth-century debuts.

Bharata natyam's repertoire consists largely of songs written between the seventeenth and twentieth centuries. The poems of love and religious devotion that form the basis of the bharata natyam canon emerged from the musical and literary traditions of previous centuries. The sung poetic text that accompanies bharata natyam choreography rests on the conventions of *bhakti*, or devotionalism, which center on the worship of deities in personal, emotional terms. Bhakti emphasized role-playing and characterization and thus inspired a number of artistic projects, including a repertoire of dance music. The idiom of *sringara bhakti*, or devotion through eroticism, aligned sexual love and religious devotion. These idioms, which first developed in the sixth and seventh centuries CE, undergird much of today's solo choreography.

Bharata natyam's relationship to its past, however, is neither implicit nor unselfconscious.[1] Rather, twentieth-century dancers connected their performance work to that of the past through specific choices in repertoire, choreographic themes, and movement vocabulary. They referenced Sanskrit texts, Tamil literature, temple sculpture, and religious ritual, using them in divergent ways and making their engagement with the dance form's history more apparent in choreography and pedagogy than earlier dancers had done. Practitioners also put forward commentaries that outlined their understanding of bharata natyam's past as it established the aesthetic values of the present. This intentional and overt use of historical sources separated their practice from that of pre-revival performers.[2] They emphasized specific antecedents for the dance genre and downplayed others, decisions that aligned with their discussions of bharata natyam's identity, function, and rightful place in society. The histories they proposed, as the selection of certain elements of practice and cultural influences to the exclusion of others, varied depending on their attention to distant or recent origins, to local, regional, or national traditions, and to concerns of gender and class. Different understandings of bharata natyam's past therefore dovetailed with divergent politics of representation.

Moreover, despite commonalities between bharata natyam and earlier practice, present-day performance reflects changes in performance content and context. Some dancers in the twentieth century transformed the choreography's style of rendition, extending lines out into space and augmenting the angularity of positions. Others broadened its floor patterns, traveling across more of the performance area than sadir dancers did in order to suit the larger proscenium theaters of the twentieth century. Similarly, some performers amplified the facial expressions of the abhinaya, debating the use of theatrical versus naturalistic expression and foregrounding the use of full-body pantomime, again with the aim of rendering the expressions legible to a less proximate audience.

Repertoire has also changed. Even the most traditional choreography is not completely fixed: it transforms in the process of its transmission. A conventional bharata natyam piece consists of a compilation of phrases set to the music of a dance style's customary repertoire. Dance teachers arrange material learned from their mentors but assembled according to their own decisions. Historically, nattuvanars set choreography but did not dance publicly; dancers performed but did not create new works themselves. Instead, dancers improvised decisions in performance, choices that sometimes found their way into a set version of a piece.

The twentieth century offered further opportunities for change as dancers moved between performing and teaching. Nineteenth-century practice adhered to a gendered division of labor in which devadasis danced and their nattuvanars taught; twentieth-century dancers took up these two tasks simultaneously. This allowed dancers to transition from performance into arrangement and composition. Opportunities for creation included the crafting of items within the conventional margam genres and the choreography of innovative pieces with new structures. For example, dancers devised material that fit within the solo reper-

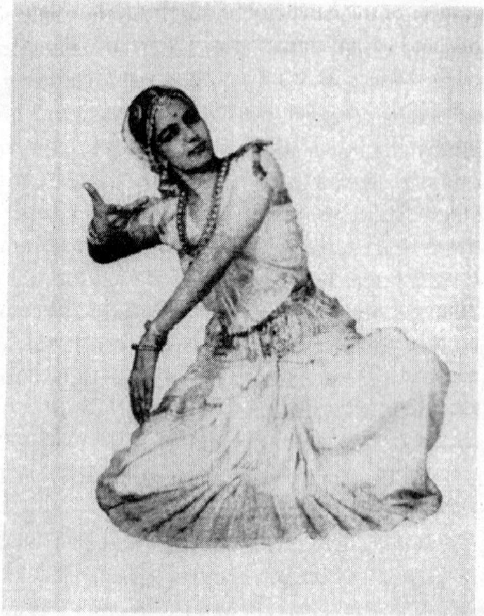

Figure 5: Rukmini Devi in the twentieth-century bharata natyam costume. Courtesy of Jerome Robbins Dance Division, The New York Public Library for the Performing Arts, Astor, Lenox and Tilden Foundations.

toire but that relied upon non-dance music or out-of-circulation choreography from the past. Likewise, practitioners commissioned music and created pieces outside conventional genres, choreographing ensemble works and evening-length pieces based on the bharata natyam movement vocabulary.

The previous century has also seen changes, in Susan Foster's (1986) terms, to the elements that frame performance. The use of the term bharata natyam as the sole appellation for the dance form is a twentieth-century development. The now-traditional bharata natyam costume developed through Rukmini Devi's and Ram Gopal's experiments with concert attire in the 1930s (Ramnarayan 1984b: 28; Khokar 2004: 37). The context of performance has also changed. Devadasis danced in a number of settings, including courts, temples, and public festivals, as well as in the homes of patrons. By contrast, post-revival dancers restricted their concerts to the urban proscenium theaters until the 1980s, when organizers began presenting festivals in temples.

Despite these changes, most dancers who define their work as classical bharata natyam concur that a sense of continuity should undergird choreographic endeavors. However, ideas of authenticity, tradition, classicism, and history do not automatically generate or rely upon consensus. Rather, each of these concepts has a range of possible definitions that performers draw from and deploy in different ways. Individual dancers diverge in their understanding of what the most important aspect of the dance form's history is, how best to express allegiance to that history, and what elements of dance practice should be maintained or revivified. Through these contrasting definitions of classicism and history, bharata natyam dancers also put forth their own ideas of creativity and expressivity. Not only did twentieth-century bharata natyam undergo some particularly notable changes, but, at the same time, dancers' appeals to the past were evident. Explanations for this apparent paradox are tied to the early twentieth century and to the move to recontextualize that era's performance practice.

This chapter draws out the different definitions of tradition and the accompanying, contrasting versions of history that performers proposed, locating these varied points of view in the social, political, and artistic perspectives of each dancer. I argue that dancers relied upon views of creativity that supported their understanding of bharata natyam's past and illustrate the tensions between individual contribution and allegiance to tradition that characterize twentieth-century bharata natyam, indicating that they are mutually constituting rather than that they work in opposition. The pages that follow trace a genealogy of histories, indicating the different identities that performers crafted for the dance form through reference to its past.

The Anti-Nautch Movement, Textual Orientalism, and Dance Orientalism

Sadir, the solo, female dance form associated with the literary and musical traditions of southern India, was performed by devadasis, courtesans and ritual officiants dedicated to temple and court service. Devadasis never married but lived instead in female-headed households with their grandmothers, mothers, and children. The ritual confirming their entry into temple service paralleled the wedding ceremony for other women: devadasis married the presiding deity of their temple. They were then considered *nityasumangali*, ever-auspicious women (Kersenboom-Story 1987). Because auspiciousness—the spiritual power associated with domestic stability and good fortune—and social standing in mainstream Hindu society depended on a woman's status as a wife with a living husband, a devadasi inhabited a unique position: her auspicious state, linked to an immortal spouse, endured lifelong. Despite this marriage to the deity, devadasis did not remain sexually abstinent. Rather, they entered into liaisons with men, initially selected by the senior women of their household, who became their patrons. These affiliations were nondomestic: they kept separate homes and did not perform household tasks for patrons. Children remained with their devadasi mother.

Devadasis trained in dance and music and, unlike most other women of their time, learned to read and write. They traveled about freely in the outside world, which contemporaneous elite women did not, although, in some cases, women so dedicated to the deity had to remain in the city (Marglin 1985: 33). They received a salary from the temple or court and supplemented this income with grants earned for particular performances. In devadasi households, unlike in most other Hindu families, parents preferred girl children to boys, because females continued the hereditary occupation and performed key domestic rituals. Elder women controlled financial and other decisions in these households.

Nonetheless, social and economic dependence on men curtailed the relative freedoms that these women exercised. Although they received a salary, devadasis relied on their patrons for nonessentials. In addition, devadasi households entertained lavishly, which depleted even substantial resources (Srinivasan 1985: 1872). Their presence moreover contributed to a sexual double standard in which society allowed elite men both wives and mistresses while restricting most women to lifelong monogamy. Devadasis' autonomous income in the form of a salary and even their land holdings depended on their remaining in service and upholding the system by initiating their daughters into the devadasi office (Anandhi 1991: 740).

Marginal but respected, receiving their own income but tied to temple or court service and deriving luxury items from patrons, devadasis were ambiguous figures in pre- and early colonial Tamil society. Anti-nautch agitations complicated the devadasis' status further because they brought temple women to the fore of a controversy over the status of women and "native" cultural practices. This movement, begun in South India in 1892, mobilized against the dedication of women and girls as devadasis to ritual service and against their related performance practice. Nautch is an anglicization of *nach*, a Hindi word for dance. Hence, the movement identified itself as an "anti-dance" movement, even as it focused on the status of women and the social structures around ritual dedication. Anti-nautch activists attempted to eradicate courtesanship by abolishing the hereditary offices of temple and court service and by eliminating the performance of sadir. The ostensible prurience of the dance, reformers maintained, supported a system that institutionalized prostitution; moreover, courtesanship had cultivated a lascivious dance form.

By contrast, revivalists—nationalist activists invested in maintaining ancient Hindu traditions—defended the devadasi system. Unlike reformers, who relied at least in part on Victorian feminism, revivalists celebrated indigenous cultural practices and upheld the social status quo (Sangari 1989). The nationalist-revivalist camp set the stage for bharata natyam's refiguration in the 1930s by locating evidence of cultural accomplishment in precolonial Indian practices. Some revivalists focused their attention specifically on dance, positing that indigenous classical forms were cultural treasures that would contribute to national pride.

The devadasis of Madras presidency fit easily into neither reformist nor revivalist camps. They collectively opposed anti-dedication legislation on both material and aesthetic grounds, agitating for the right to retain their hereditary offices and their livelihood. Like the revivalists, devadasis argued that temple dedication and dance practice need not necessarily result in courtesanship (Arudra 1986–87a: 19). Further, they maintained that the legislation itself would encourage prostitution in their communities because it left women without a source of income (Jordan 1989: 263–75).

Although anti-nautch activists did not secure legislation against dedication until 1947, by the early years of the twentieth century they had eroded public support for dance and pushed sadir to the margins of social life. During the first two decades of the twentieth century, sadir remained stigmatized, and respectable elites frowned upon its performance. Although still practiced, the dance form had fallen from favor.[3] The eradication of patronage and of public approval displaced sadir, leaving it without a clear social or aesthetic function and with minimal economic support. Anti-nautch agitations altered dance practice as much as they did ritual protocol and domestic arrangements.

A new generation of practitioners, most of them descended from non-devadasi communities, turned to solo South Indian dance in the 1920s and 1930s, bringing it to the modern urban concert stage. As they did so, they strove to salvage a disparaged and displaced form. The anti-nautch attempt to excise sadir from public life left bharata natyam without an immediate, visible, and respectable precedent for its appearance in the theaters of the cities. The anti-nautch movement's discrediting of dance meant that the revival's performers needed to justify their practice of the dance form. Performers responded to such criticisms by validating their decisions to study and perform bharata natyam through recourse to history, foregrounding elements of the past both choreographically and discursively. They strove to avoid the stigma that afflicted the devadasi legacy by either circumventing or reclaiming the recent past and justified their performance of bharata natyam by linking it to other artistic and ritual practices. This look to the past sparked debates over the history of dance. In sanctioning contemporary performance through reference to historical sources for choreographic decisions, dancers responded not only to anti-nautch criticism but also to Orientalist thought.[4]

Colonialists justified imperial rule by claiming that their imposition of an alien government and economy reformed colonized societies and brought them in line with European post-Enlightenment values. Colonizers argued that theirs was a "civilizing mission," intended to uplift those they ruled by freeing them from their own oppressive practices. Imperial rulers claimed to bring civilization to an otherwise degraded populace. They criticized "the East" for remaining fettered by tradition while "the West" embraced change and vitality. At the same time, colonial Orientalists valorized ancient textual traditions.[5] This celebration of the subcontinent's high-culture past, however, did not compel Orientalists to reject the colonial rescue narrative. Orientalist scholars reconciled the two perspectives and maintained that contemporaneous India was the attenuated remnant of an illustrious civilization, with the authentic India remaining in the past rather than existing in the present.

Formed through an unequal but dialogic exchange between Brahman informants and English and German scholars, Orientalist writings privileged the voices of elites, their cultural and literary products, and their ritual practices (Inden 1990; Ramaswamy 1997: 27, 38–39). The discovery that Sanskrit, as a progenitor of the Indo-European language group, linked India to Europe accelerated this glorification of India's past and its canonical texts. Orientalists further maintained that civilization inhered in classical traditions and, tautologically, that "classicism" provided evidence of civilization. They located India's "civilized" legacy in the hegemonic Sanskrit language and literature and in the communities that maintained them. For Orientalists, India's greatness lay doubly in the past: because civilization required "classicism," by definition rooted in history, and because invasions and political corruption had, they maintained, diluted India's access to its classical traditions and, hence, its civilizational status.

As the historian Sumathi Ramaswamy (1997) argues, the logic of colonialism depended upon this putative cultural deficit for its moral justification. The independence movement then required that nationalists counter the premise of native inferiority by supplying evidence of indigenous accomplishment. Nationalists replaced the narrative of the civilizing mission with one that celebrated local cultural products and represented them as equal to, if not better than, those of the colonizer. Through a process that Ramaswamy labels a "nostalgia for civilization," nationalists and regionalists struggled against the colonial condemnation of Indian society and strove to reconstruct the merits of its past in the present.

When, in the 1930s, a new generation of dancers took to the concert stage under the auspices of nationalism, they faced a dilemma: how to celebrate the heritage that made India unique while contesting colonialist charges of stagnation. Performers resolved this quandary by proposing specific origins for bharata natyam that accommodated a validating classical culture while also highlighting the creativity that inhered in the form. They argued that contemporary, innovative agendas found expression in bharata natyam and that traditionalism did not preclude originality. Practitioners embodied this dual agenda when they posited historical origins that supported their choreographic choices.

This imperative, split between originality and historicity, surfaced in choreography in response to the dance form's intersection not only with colonialism and nationalism but also with global discourses of artistic originality (Allen 1998; Coorlawala 1996; Srinivasan 2003). European and North American premodern and early modern dancers represented choreography as an autonomous, creative venture that addressed serious intellectual and philosophical themes rather than merely providing entertainment. The idea of dance as "high art" rather than as a diversion in turn inflected the recontextualization of bharata natyam. For instance, a 1938 newspaper article credited the new seriousness that the modern-

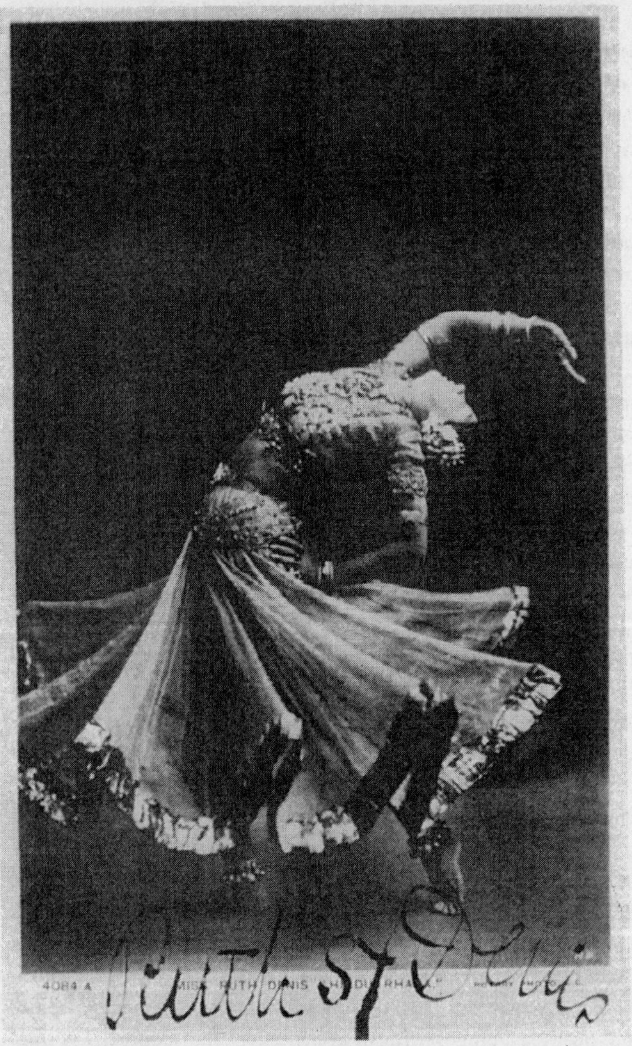

Figure 6: Ruth St. Denis in *Radha.* © V & A Images/Victoria and Albert Museum.

dance movement had ascribed to dance with the support offered to the Michigan-born classical Indian dancer Ragini Devi during her European tours ("The Dance in Indian Sagas," 1938). Moreover, a number of dancers who laid claim to innovation in dance, including the modern-dance forerunner Ruth St. Denis, the ballerina and choreographer Anna Pavlova, and the Indian modernist Uday Shankar, played a role in the bharata natyam revival, urging attention to "forgotten" Indian arts while also signaling the importance of creative invention. The dancers of the bharata natyam revival deployed this ideology of originality, and its accompanying notions of interiority, inspiration, and the concept of autonomous art, to challenge Orientalist claims of stasis while also differentiating their endeavors from devadasi practice.[6]

At the same time, however, an Orientalist emphasis on "Eastern tradition," in dance and in public culture generally, colored bharata natyam's intersection with global dance modernism. Early modernists and interpretive dancers relied on classical dance as the foil that highlighted their own creative ventures (Chatterjea 2004a; Srinivasan 2003). The same international figures who prompted inquiry into the solo Indian dance forms sought out practices that would corroborate their understandings of "the East" as spiritual and steeped in ancient tradition. For these reasons, as well as because of the success of institutions such as the Music Academy and Kalakshetra in rendering classical dance visible, twentieth-century viewers came to expect markers of continuity in Indian dance and rejected invention for its own sake. By mid-century, international and Indian audiences privileged classical Indian dances over modernist ones: for example, Shankar's cross-cultural fusions enjoyed popularity in the 1920s and 1930s but later incurred criticism for their eclecticism.[7] The revival's bharata natyam dancers differentiated their projects from more experimental works such as Shankar's not only by upholding continuity in dance technique and repertoire, but also by pointing to historical precedent for the innovations that they made.

Revival-era practitioners contended with local economic upheavals as well as with global artistic epistemologies. Initially, imperialism destabilized royal authority and removed the economic structures that supported classical Indian arts. Anti-nautch activists subsequently criticized the colonial government for supporting dance performance, while an independent state had not yet emerged to formulate its own arts policy. These shifts in political systems and in public perception of performance affected sadir directly, because it cut off financial support for Thanjavur's devadasis (Meduri 1996). The performers who entered the dance arena in the 1930s therefore depended on *sabhas* (private, voluntary arts organizations) and, post-1947, on government agencies for their support. The shift from a feudal system to a postcolonial market economy left a new generation of performers with increased freedom and decreased stability. Although the independent Indian government introduced socialist initiatives, such as land reform and state ownership of large industry, it also retained features of a capitalist economy. As Janet Wolff (1987) argues, the economic precariousness of a capitalist art market fosters the idea of "autonomous art" by releasing practitioners from the need to please patrons and pushing them instead to compete with one another, so that they have a vested interest in proving their uniqueness. Moreover, when artistic practice no longer restricts itself to hereditary groups, the number of performers can increase. Even when a government funds artistic endeavors, as in India, performers compete against a host of others in a similar position and therefore need to establish the singularity of their work. Private organizations depend on memberships and other kinds of individual or corporate contributions. This scarcity of resources in relation to the number of artists dictates the selection of some performers over others according to particular criteria.

However, the social and political investments of the late colonial and early postcolonial period complicated an economic situation that encouraged individuality. Government agencies and private cultural organizations consolidated themselves around nationalist or regionalist agendas. These forms of sponsorship encouraged dancers' performance work to align, in some way, with the outlook of the funding body, often through reference to past practice and its relationship to present-day communities. At the same time, they required evidence of uniqueness in order to differentiate between dancers. Such organizations, finding themselves in the position of choosing one dancer over others, sought evidence of both exceptionality and continuity.

These two apparently competing agendas—originality and traditionalism—thus developed in reaction to the political forces that inflected the refiguration of solo South Indian dance as a concert art. Twentieth-century dancers deployed markers of both historicity and creativity in performance and in their commentaries on the dance practice, relying upon and resisting the assumptions of the colonial moment in which bharata natyam appeared as a stage art. Practitioners articulated these concerns by staging their understanding of the dance form's past in both performance and verbal form. The rest of the chapter follows the genealogy through which this dance form came to embody both traditionalism and originality.

Originality and Origin in the Revival

E. Krishna Iyer (1897–1968), a Tamil Brahman lawyer, was one initiator of the multiple transformations that bharata natyam underwent during the revival.[8] In 1923, the twenty-six-year-old sought out dance training from the renowned performer Madurantakam Jagadambal in order to prepare for a role in *Malavikagnimitra*, a Sanskrit play. He segued into solo performance when the dance guru A. P. Natesa Iyer heard of his abilities and offered to train him in sadir.[9] At the urging of his mentor, E. Krishna Iyer set out to restore sadir to its rightful place in public life, undertaking this mission through concerts of conventional dance pieces, or margam items. Iyer assumed devadasi attire and, through both his appearance and his performance skill, convinced audiences that he was not only a woman but also a hereditary dancer. Conjoining these performances with lectures on the aesthetic value of sadir, he toured throughout southern India.

Subsequently, Iyer entered the political arena as a nationalist activist, turning his attention away from performance and toward arts promotion and criticism

(Gaston 1996: 93; Raman and Ramachandran 1984b: 29). As joint secretary of the reception committee, Iyer, along with two colleagues, organized the 1927 All India Music Conference that accompanied the Madras meeting of the Indian National Congress. In 1928, when the Music Academy was formally established, Iyer retained his role as joint secretary. Subsequently imprisoned by the colonial government for his role in nationalist agitations, Iyer urged his fellow activist prisoners to support dance. Upon his release, he persuaded the Music Academy officers to promote sadir. The academy board made a trailblazing move when they agreed to his proposal and included a performance by the Kalyani daughters, the devadasi dancers Rajalakshmi and Jeevaratnam, in its 1931 concert series. Disinterest and ambivalence met this first attempt, but a subsequent performance by the dancers was well attended.

Iyer also distinguished himself in the dance field by directly challenging the anti-nautch campaign of Muttulakshmi Reddy. Reddy, herself from a devadasi family,[10] was a medical doctor and feminist activist who campaigned for anti-dedication legislation and the abolition of temple dance. In 1930, she authored the Madras Devadasis Prevention of Dedication bill in order to free dedicated women from their dependence on ritual service and sexual patronage and ideally to encourage them into conventional, monogamous marriages. This, she believed, would also eradicate the stigma on the devadasi community (Nair 1994: 3164). When sadir appeared in two public functions in 1932, Reddy voiced her complaints in letters to two English-language dailies, *The Mail* and *The Hindu* (Arudra 1986–87a: 19). Iyer countered Reddy's arguments by defending the aesthetic value of the dance and the role it could play in the cultural life of the nation. The two debated the validity of devadasi dance through a volley of letters until the editor of *The Hindu* discontinued their dialogue. Iyer then wrote an open letter to the president of the Madras Music Academy requesting that the academy's board raise the issue at their annual meeting (Arudra 1986–87a: 19). The academy sponsored a debate on December 28, 1932, circulating a resolution in advance that Iyer had proposed in favor of dance performance and patronage. Musicians, scholars, and critics came forward in support of sadir, rejecting anti-nautch claims in speeches that emphasized the dance form's aesthetic and social merits, and eventually passed a resolution in favor of the dance form. This resolution was also instrumental in confirming the change of the dance form's name from sadir to bharata natyam.[11]

The term bharata natyam sanctioned the form, distancing it from devadasi words for dance, such as sadir, *dasi attam*, and *chinna mela*. The name also carried etymological associations that validated the form by invoking the *Natyasastra*, Indian classical music, and music theory. The term natya moreover connotes a multigenre theater form rather than solo dance, linking bharata natyam to pan-Indian dramatic traditions and distancing it from the solo performance of devadasi dancers. These connotations for bharata natyam, in contrast to the

Tamil devadasi names, carry the prestige of the Sanskrit language and suggest elite, pan-Indian associations.

The Music Academy prompted another strategy of the revival—the "textualisation of dance" (Srinivasan 1983)—in 1930, when it included an article in the first issue of its journal by V. Venkatarama Sharma, who argued that bharata natyam accorded with the tenets of the *Natyasastra* (Arudra 1986–87a: 18). Subsequently, the organization fueled the revival not only by legitimizing bharata natyam through activism and critical inquiry, but also by presenting concerts by the most influential dancers of the period during its annual festival season in December and January. In addition to the recitals by the Kalyani daughters in 1931 and 1933, they presented a 1932 performance by the renowned devadasi dancer Mylapore Gowri Ammal, who in turn influenced both Rukmini Devi and Balasaraswati. During the first part of the decade, the academy sponsored presentations by other devadasi performers; by the late 1930s, adolescent Brahman girls were appearing on the academy's stage. This foray of high-caste, middle-class young women into performance and its support by the Music Academy cemented the gains of the revival and affirmed the respectability of bharata natyam. The revivalist goal of legitimizing dance by involving high-status women in public performances was realized.

Rukmini Devi (1904–1986), who was in the audience of a 1935 Music Academy dance recital, extended this validation process through her efforts in performance, pedagogy, and composition. Rukmini Devi's first entries into the Madras public sphere came in the 1920s not through dance, but through nationalist activism and theosophy, an eclectic, transnational religious movement. Devi hailed from a Tamil Brahman family with a background in Sanskrit scholarship and music; her father was a member of the theosophical movement (Ramnarayan 1984a: 19–20).

As an adolescent, Devi came under the tutelage of Annie Besant, an English theosophist and proponent of Indian nationalism. Besant, though British, served as president of the Indian National Congress from 1917 to 1918. Her politics drew on the Orientalist-nationalist underpinnings of her religious community: for her, India's right to independence arose directly out of its value as a great civilization with an ancient history, rooted in Sanskrit and Upanishadic Hinduism (Allen 1997). Besant's position rested upon Orientalist and nationalist discourse and thus contributed to, in the historian Sumathi Ramaswamy's (1997) terms, "neo-Hindu" Indian nationalism. According to Ramaswamy, neo-Hindu activists celebrated the merits of contemporary India as descended from the glorious traditions of an ancient past (26–27). Rukmini Devi espoused political beliefs similar to Besant's and promoted the Theosophical Society's social causes. Like Iyer, Rukmini Devi began her artistic career in the field of drama. She participated in (and later directed) theatrical productions at the Theosophical Society, including politically inflected performances. Her activism and theater work, combined with her marriage to the English theosophist George Arundale, threw her into the spotlight of Madras's public arena.

Fortuitous circumstances channeled Rukmini Devi's artistic and political interests into dance. In 1928, while touring Australia and Southeast Asia on Theosophical Society business, Rukmini Devi met Anna Pavlova, whose dancing she had seen and admired in Bombay (Ramnarayan 1984a: 29; Sarada 1985: 40). Pavlova encouraged Rukmini Devi to learn dance, offering to provide instruction herself and arranging for her to study with her soloist Cleo Nordi until Pavlova could join her in London. Although the ballerina died before Rukmini Devi could train with her, Pavlova left a lasting impact by suggesting a way for Devi to combine her devotion to dance, spirituality, and nationalism. Pavlova had installed ballet as a "high art" and shifted public opinion of the form. She likewise encouraged her friend to "revive the art of [her] own country" (quoted in Ramnarayan 1984a: 29), a statement that inspired Devi to seek out training with traditional practitioners of sadir in Madras. In 1935, at the suggestion of E. Krishna Iyer, she attended a performance at the Music Academy, approached devadasi dancers, and finally met Mylapore Gowri Ammal, who accepted her as a student. She later pursued training under Meenakshisundaram Pillai, a guru of the Isai Vellala caste, a community from which most devadasis and nattuvanars came.[12]

In December 1935, Rukmini Devi gave her debut concert for the Theosophical Society's anniversary celebrations. Although this performance was not a formal arangetram,[13] it launched Rukmini Devi's dance career. Her determination to dance stirred up a furor among the anti-nautch elites of Madras, and, according to the theosophist Barbara Sellon, some of those invited boycotted her debut performance but many other curious onlookers appeared, swelling the audience to almost a thousand (Sellon, cited in Ramnarayan 1984b: 21). Rukmini Devi's performance won over her detractors and convinced remaining skeptics of the aesthetic value of the form. A month later, in January 1936, Devi founded Kalakshetra, an institution housed on Theosophical Society grounds where she provided students with training in bharata natyam, *kathakali*, and Carnatic music. Rukmini Devi's status as a middle-class Brahman woman and as a respected public figure, combined with the arguments she put forth in favor of the dance, accelerated the bharata natyam revival and convinced a wider public of the legitimacy of the dance form.

Tanjore Balasaraswati (1918–1984) entered the dance field from a position distinct from that of either E. Krishna Iyer or Rukmini Devi. One of the first dancers to appear at the Music Academy, she was also one of the only devadasis to continue performing through the revival and beyond. She thus bridged a gap between devadasi and higher-caste dancers (Allen 1997: 64–65; Gaston 1996: 81; Singer 1958: 374). Balasaraswati came from a Madras-based family of musicians descended from performers of the Thanjavur court. Her mother, Jayammal, and her grandmother, the legendary veena player Dhanammal, trained her in music and music appreciation from a young age. As a small child, Balasaraswati visited her neighbor Mylapore Gowri Ammal and imitated her dancing. The latter suggested that Balasaraswati learn dance, a proposal Jayammal and Dhanammal initially rejected. Eventually Dhanammal gave her permission, and Balasaraswati began, at the age of four, to study with Kandappa Pillai, a nattuvanar who, like his student, came from a family with several generations of involvement in the Thanjavur court music and dance milieu.

Balasaraswati presented her arangetram in 1925. In spite of anti-nautch pressure, her debut replicated devadasi precedent as it took place in the Ammanakshi temple in Kanchipuram. She gave her first concert at the Music Academy in 1933, initiating a long-standing relationship with the institution. The concert also brought Balasaraswati to national renown: Uday Shankar attended and was so captivated by her dancing that he requested a repeat performance. He invited Balasaraswati to join his company but, on Jayammal's advice, she refused, concerned that Shankar's experiments would dilute the classicism of their family's tradition (Arudra 1986–87a: 20, 1986–87b: 25; Raman and Ramachandran 1984a: 28). However, Haren Ghosh, a friend of Shankar's and an impresario, was also in the audience. He arranged Balasaraswati's first concert outside of southern India, in Calcutta, which led to other concerts in North India and thus bolstered her national, and eventually international, reputation.

These performances, in North India and globally, both fostered Balasaraswati's career and furthered the gains of the revival more generally.[14] Although Balasaraswati identified herself as a traditionalist who fought the tide of change, she nonetheless, through her skill as a performer and her standing as a hereditary practitioner, contributed to bharata natyam's new status as an urban, concert art form. She brought a sense of continuity to the recently recontextualized form as she argued in favor of maintaining its key aesthetic features. Although she fought moves to "improve" the dance by aligning it with the premises of aesthetic theory, she nonetheless supported the burgeoning respectability of the form by noting parallels between it and the dance practices described in Tamil literature and Sanskrit theory.

Rukmini Devi and Balasaraswati differed not only in their background and their initial performance experiences, but also in their approaches to bharata natyam. Indeed, at first glance, each of these two dancers seems to represent one of the apparently competing tendencies of creativity versus allegiance to tradition. Devi enjoys pride of place as the first modern bharata natyam choreographer, while Balasaraswati inspires devotion as a purist who fought the tide of history. Devi developed original choreography for solo conventional dance items, created new margam items, choreographed for classical songs that had not previously operated as dance accompaniment, and created ensemble works.[15] Balasaraswati, although she performed in and occasionally created ensemble pieces, achieved renown primarily as a performer within the solo margam, with national and international audiences praising her skill in evoking dramatic scenarios through structured improvisation. The dancers' aims likewise differed according to their contrasting priorities and perspectives on the dance form. Devi strove to salvage bharata natyam and to erase its stigma, purifying it while also aligning it with modern aesthetic values.[16] Balasaraswati sought to uphold a tradition that she saw as continuous, aiming to protect bharata natyam from alteration.

These two practitioners also provided divergent accounts of bharata natyam's history and its ideal state. They described the most significant traditional values of the form as emerging out of disparate historical moments. For Devi, allegiance to past precedent meant recapturing the features of the multigenre "total theater" of Sanskrit drama (Peterson 1998: 58) and resurrecting these values in the present. Balasaraswati, by contrast, portrayed as traditional the repertory and concert-order principles laid down by the nineteenth-century Thanjavur Quartet and transmitted through an oral tradition of devadasi dancers and their nattuvanar mentors.

Each dancer likewise situated creativity in a different aspect of choreographic practice. Devi located artistic expression in the composition of new works, while Balasaraswati found aesthetic inspiration in the opportunities for expressivity offered by improvised sections of a dance performance. Devi undertook new choreographic ventures that, she maintained, accessed "the spirit of the traditional methods" (in Ramnarayan 1984c: 29), while Balasaraswati believed that inherited repertoire provided ample scope for the exploitation of imagination (Bannerjee 1988: 39). These dancers put forth two divergent arguments about the relationship between creativity and continuity.

However, although they defined both tradition and individual expression differently, Devi and Balasaraswati shared the basic premise that bharata natyam could best express originality through fidelity to the past. Although each referred to contrasting historical moments and different aspects of performance, both foregrounded the importance of tradition, identifying quality in bharata natyam as the preservation of fundamental elements of an originary dance practice. Both found creativity within classicism rather than in experimentation for its own sake. Their work therefore met at a crucial point: each located originality within continuity. Devi and Balasaraswati proposed contrasting versions of the dance form's identity while sharing a basic understanding about it. For both, the dance form's history remained an index of its aesthetic quality.

After a brief stint as an interpretive dancer,[17] Rukmini Devi pursued a short but influential career as a solo bharata natyam artist. Her most significant contributions, however, came not through performance, but through the revision of pedagogical methods and the composition of new works. She introduced changes to instruction and performance, suggesting that these developments neither broke from tradition nor replicated it. Similarly, she infused bharata natyam with new choreographic structures and themes that expressed the values of traditional practice while not necessarily mimicking its form.[18] Through these projects, Devi conjoined two agendas of originality and allegiance to the past into a single style of choreography.

When she founded the Kalakshetra institution, Devi revamped bharata natyam training by introducing the idea of a dedicated dance school where students learned in formal dance classes. This approach contrasted with the ongoing learning process that constituted the traditional *gurukula* arrangement, in which a student lives with the teacher to pursue long-term immersion in dance study through both formal lessons and informal tutelage.[19] The gurukula or *gurusishya* system is informal in that students learn not only through classes with the teacher but also through observation and, eventually, by teaching the mentor's junior students. The pace of instruction is individualized in this system: each student proceeds at her own rate. There are no exams, grades, or official markers of progress (except for the arangetram), and instruction is continuous, not marked by entry into new levels or by a graduation out of tutelage. The student provides domestic and other assistance in lieu of payment.

Despite these fluid qualities, gurusishya teaching methods are both tightly organized and authoritative. Gurukula instruction follows a standardized pattern in that a student acquires the basic movement units, or *adavus*, in a set order, proceeding to new material only after mastering the earlier. When students proceed to repertoire, the process replicates the concert order, with students learning a *jatisvaram* after completing *alarippu* and so forth. Students learn through direct practice and imitation, not through questioning or explanation. According to traditional gurusishya protocol, the student dancer learns under one mentor only. The young dancer embodies the aesthetic values of a mentor's artistic lineage by replicating the teacher's repertoire and style of rendition (Ananya 1996); only after a student has trained long enough to internalize these priorities does she move on to improvisation.

The Kalakshetra school, by contrast, standardized the means through which students learned dance, providing them with a syllabus complete with grade levels and exams. Rukmini Devi thus created an institution based on modern models of education, ensuring that teachers gave instruction in a consistent manner and guaranteeing that students gain the type and amount of information appropriate to their level, a project that, as Uttara Coorlawala argues, aligned bharata natyam training with the British dance syllabus system (1996: 67). Rukmini Devi also developed a system in which student dancers learn from different Kalakshetra teachers at various times in their training. In doing so, she encouraged her pupils to replace the more conventional loyalty to a single teacher with a fidelity to the school.

Kalakshetra also provides instruction in Sanskrit aesthetic theory alongside practical lessons. At each level, students memorize appropriate verses on and categories of dramaturgical classification (Sarada 1985: 21; Coorlawala 1996: 66). Al-

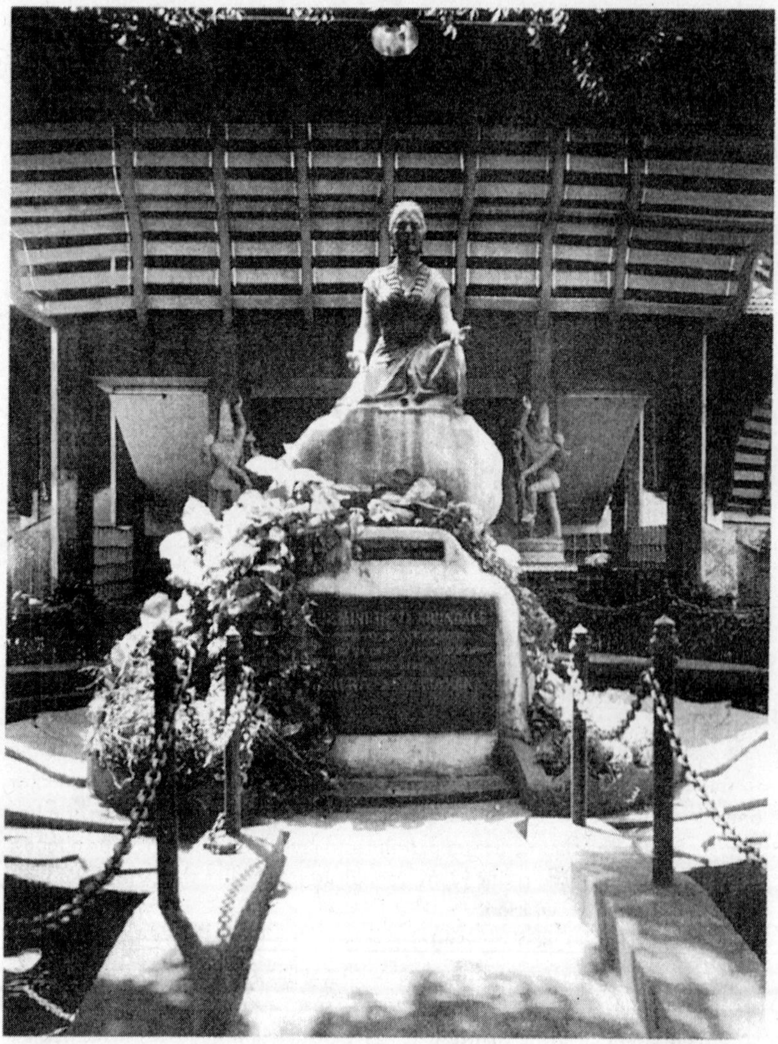

Figure 7: Statue of Rukmini Devi in front of the Kalakshetra Theatre. Photograph by author.

though rooted in ancient texts, this transformation of pedagogical methods relied on modern values: Rukmini Devi provided training in aesthetic theory so that students would understand the reasons for what they did. She encouraged students to investigate the theoretical underpinnings of classical dance practice and not merely replicate what their teachers imparted. This move democratized dance instruction by giving students greater agency in the learning process and by offering them the opportunity for increased knowledge (Gaston 1996: 125; Meduri 1996: 366–72; Ramnarayan 1984a: 22). Through this process, Devi helped dancers of subsequent generations to create an educated, authoritative position in relation to the form.

Rukmini Devi brought an egalitarian angle to dance training by rejecting a need for obedience. At the same time, however, the loyalty to the school that it cultivated reveals a modern concern with individuals internalizing rules so that dancers discipline themselves. There is a parallel here between embodying the rules of dance, as part of dance education, and the Foucauldian (1979) paradigm of modernity in which citizens internalize discipline rather than experiencing it as submission to an outside force. Through such attention to classical principles, Kalakshetra dancers inherited a modern attention to repeatability (Franko 1989) in place of the historical priority given to the imprint of a specific mentor. This method also encouraged students to incorporate the values of the Sanskrit texts so that they developed a greater loyalty to classicism than they might have if they received instruction without theoretical justification.

Rukmini Devi not only systematized the means through which teachers imparted material, but also standardized the performance of movement to make it more consistent from one dancer to the next. In lieu of the stylistic traces associated with individual instructors that characterize the gurusishya system, Rukmini Devi developed a style emblematic of the institution as a whole. She preserved the steps and dynamics of the Pandanallur tradition in which she trained, but she also included, at first, ballet exercises added to render the adavus more accurate (Sarada 1985: 20). Rukmini Devi used ballet training to influence the stylistic rendition of units of movement rather than to alter the vocabulary itself, augmenting an existing classical attention to shape and angular line. Devi privileged precision and accuracy in choreography, especially in nritta, the rhythmic aspect of performance. She highlighted the Pandanallur style's emphasis on spatiality (Coorlawala 1996: 68; Meduri 1996: 334): the extension of the limbs in clean, clear lines typifies the adavus of the Kalakshetra style. She thus emphasized geometry over rhythmic counterpoint. At the same time, however, Devi also cultivated rhythmic precision in her dancers, foregrounding less the mathematical complexity typical of Carnatic music than a metrical correspondence between footwork and hand, arm, and upper-body movement. Thus, she created a Kalakshetra style that was exact, precise, and articulate.

By instructing student dancers to produce defined movements apprehended through uniform means, Rukmini Devi generated a pool of performers uniquely suited to group choreography.[20] Her Kalakshetra institution required such dancers because she elevated ensemble work to a new level of importance. Over the course of a forty-year choreographic career (1944–84), she composed twenty-five dance dramas, of which seven were reconstructions and eighteen were completely new works based on the Indian literary canon (Ramnarayan 1984c: 38; Sarada

1985: 62–212). She based these new works on mythological themes, Sanskrit plays, and Tamil dance drama forms, including the all-male Brahman theatrical form *bhagavata mela natakam* and the eighteenth- and nineteenth-century multigenre *kuravanji*. She took responsibility for aspects of composition that ranged from the development of scenarios, commissioning scores, and setting the movement to dancing in pieces herself, at least initially.

Devi began her foray into ensemble choreography with the reconstruction in 1944 of an out-of-circulation Tamil dance drama, the *Kutrala Kuravanji* (Ramnarayan 1984c: 27–28; Sarada 1985: 40–42; Peterson 1998: 39–40, 57–63). She composed the dance sequences and employed the musician Veena Krishnamachariar to develop the melody of the songs based on the existing poetic text. Despite her interest in the values, not the form, of historical genres, she conducted extensive research in order to faithfully reconstitute the dance.[21] Although Devi had the option of staging *Sarabendra Bupala Kuravanji*, the only dance drama that devadasis continued to perform at the Thanjavur temple, she decided not to do so because of, among other things, the drama's praise of a human king rather than a god (Sarada 1985: 40; Ramnarayan 1984c: 27; Peterson 1998: 59) and its frank eroticism (Peterson 1998: 59–60).

This decision to stage a work neither in the current repertoire nor danced within recent memory inaugurated Rukmini Devi's role as a choreographer. She went on to achieve recognition for the composition of ensemble works accompanied by commissioned scores. Her longest-lasting impact on the dance field came through her innovative authorship of new material as well as through the transformations she made to dance pedagogy. She exercised creativity primarily through the composition of new works rather than by reinterpreting conventional ones.

That Rukmini Devi based her *Kutrala Kuravanji* on a historical work with an existing scenario, however, also aligned her inquiry with traditional practice. Although her decision to reconstruct a kuruvanji provided an opportunity for compositional investigation, its historicity allowed her to explore older aesthetic values, which she preferred to conducting experiments for their own sake. Moreover, in this project, and within her oeuvre of dance dramas generally, Devi emphasized elements of choreography that intersected with the aesthetics of ancient Sanskrit drama as identified in dramaturgical texts (Peterson 1998). Devi's primary and most sustained attention to Sanskrit dramaturgical theory, however, treated it as an influential principle rather than as a model for composition. Sanskrit texts, especially the *Natyasastra*, provided her with inspiration, not with a set of literal guidelines.[22] In Devi's commentaries, tradition, the *sastras*, and sometimes even bharata natyam itself operate as conceptual frameworks and as "guiding spirits."

In these ways Devi began to tease apart the intertwined notions of classicism and tradition. "Classical," in general terms, denotes an adherence to a specific set of defined principles, while "traditional" suggests an unbroken, handed-down heritage. The distinction made in English between the two terms parallels that made in Indian aesthetic theory between sastra and *parampara*, or between prescriptive text and oral tradition. Although Rukmini Devi did not emphasize this distinction discursively, in practice the attention she gave to the spirit rather than the structure of older choreographies separated classical aesthetics from specific items of traditional repertoire (Mavin Khoo, personal correspondence 2003). Within her choreography, classicism emerged as a set of principles that a dancer could work with and within. She created a choreographic style that relied on the practices of the past and that valued continuity but did not demand the continual replication of form. This notion of classicism, as distinct from traditional repertoire and structure, allowed her room for creative inquiry without compromising an aesthetic that she saw as fundamental to the Indian heritage.

That Rukmini Devi both referred to and refigured classicism, through changes in pedagogy and performance protocol, supported the bharata natyam revival by further bolstering the legitimacy of the dance practice. In revivifying the values of Sanskrit drama through bharata natyam, Rukmini Devi validated her choreographic innovations through recourse to a tradition that predated the devadasi repertoire. As she saw it, then, she did not so much reconstruct bharata natyam as reclassicize it. By focusing on Sanskrit drama and ancient aesthetic theory texts, as well as by aligning specific compositional decisions with these venerable sources, Devi circumvented the recent past, thereby escaping the aspersion cast on devadasi dancers and confirming the respectability of bharata natyam.

Rukmini Devi's inquiry into classicism through her emphasis on technique also allowed her to present bharata natyam as international without capitulating to a Western aesthetic. By foregrounding the technical rather than the devotional body, she was able to position bharata natyam on a par with ballet without subjecting it to European standards. She drew out ballet's Pythagorean model (Foster 1996a: 14) and Sanskrit aesthetic theory's geometric concerns (Vatsyayan 1977: xiv)[23] through the spatial priorities of the Pandanallur style and through her own interest in technique, creating a style that examined these elements rather than simply reflecting their form by, for instance, integrating the vocabularies from European concert dance or ancient Sanskrit drama.

Rukmini Devi therefore claimed universality for bharata natyam, through features marked as Indian, establishing Indian epistemologies as equivalent to those of the West and creating a choreographic project that, as I will argue in the following section, was nationalist not only in content but also in form. Her inquiry into technique and her engagement with ballet and Sanskritic aesthetics emerged out of colonial hybridity but was not a capitulation to colonial pressure; rather, it constituted a powerful rejoinder to colonial Orientalism and its charges of stasis. Her engagement with a range of practices prefigured an international awareness within the bharata natyam field, anticipating the move by some present-day choreographers to invoke a dialogue across movement languages without blending into a global homogeneity.[24] Rukmini Devi's reformulation of bharata natyam also resisted Orientalist representations of Indian dance by standardizing training protocol and thus by integrating such post-Enlightenment concepts as rationalism and democracy into bharata natyam teaching and performance. This project challenged a colonial understanding of Indian culture as trapped in fixed traditions and restricted by autocratic and authoritative hierarchies.

The attention Devi gave to the technical body rather than a primarily devotional or even expressive one also helped her to circumvent the stigma associated with devadasi performance.[25] By emphasizing technique, she mitigated sensuality and the expression of the *sringara bhakti*—devotion through an erotic idiom—that characterized devadasi performance, neutralizing the sensuality associated with the solo dancer and the devotional repertoire. The creation of uniformly proficient performers, alongside the development of group choreography, likewise deflected attention away from the display of the individual female dancer, thereby further validating the form for middle-class women. Her concern with technique as a larger, presumably universal, standard of excellence represented an apparently neutral area of inquiry where accomplishment in dance could be distanced from devadasi performance, lifestyle, and livelihood. The importance that Devi gave to the technical, rather than ritual, dancer thus enabled her to offset a continued affiliation of the dance with the nondomestic sexuality of devadasi practitioners.

Rukmini Devi's interest in dramatic development and narrative tension likewise defused enduring associations of bharata natyam with the marginal status of devadasis. In conventional items of repertoire, the dancer portrays all individuals involved in the dramatic scenario, which commonly depicts a young woman in love, her absent male lover (equated to or compared with a god), and her friend, whom she sends as a messenger. Devi's dance dramas shifted the portrayal of emotion from the individual expressivity of a solo dancer to an action-oriented plot enacted by an ensemble. The dramatic elements of performance thus rested less on the cultivation of emotional states, including romantic love and sexual desire, than on the progression of a story from exposition through conflict to resolution. By mitigating the portrayal of individual sentiment, lifting layers of poetic reference and character portrayal off the solo dancer, Rukmini Devi's dramas resolved some of the tensions created by the erotic overtones of the solo expression of sringara bhakti.

The accompanying emphasis that Rukmini Devi gave to religion and spirituality outside sringara bhakti idioms increased the legitimacy of bharata natyam and accelerated the revival. Her dance dramas emphasized the exploits of gods and mythological heroes, shifting religious aesthetics from individual expression to a narrative encounter. She also initiated changes in stage practice by placing icons of gods onstage and offering an obeisance to the stage and the nattuvanar, thus, in Anne-Marie Gaston's terms, "reritualizing" bharata natyam (1992: 156–57). Rukmini Devi bolstered the gains of the revival by distancing the dance form's devotional expression from the intricacies of sringara bhakti to a more straightforward celebration of gods and heroes, representing the dance form's religiosity in a potentially more respectable way.

Rukmini Devi's dance dramas not only validated bharata natyam, they also increased its accessibility for a larger audience. These works trace a story line that accrues narrative force as it progresses; by contrast, traditional items of repertoire deploy a lyric mode, foregrounding an individual dramatic moment, delving into its emotional complexity, and investigating it from a number of perspectives. Devi's use of the narrative form and of the blocking of characters in the stage space and the use of full-body dramatic expression meant that the audience did not have to rely solely on their comprehension of the sung poetry and the mudras in order to understand the dance. These decisions rendered the dance dramas legible to a nonspecialist audience and thus fostered their popularity nationally and internationally.

Rukmini Devi proposed a definition of tradition that, on the one hand, validated bharata natyam. On the other hand, her recourse to the distant past legitimized change by establishing a history for bharata natyam long and encompassing enough that the dance could not have avoided transforming.[26] By arguing that she reaccessed the fundamental qualities, not the exact configuration, of a traditional practice, Devi resolved a tension between authenticity and originality. This simultaneous look to both the past and the future supported her transactions with national and global politics. Her involvement in political activism as well as her experience with narrative drama and ballet, as Indira Viswanathan Peterson (1998: 58–59) suggests, inspired Devi to reconstruct the values of an ancient, pan-Indian practice that could nonetheless accommodate new structures and themes. Her desire to salvage the form, combined with her goal of establishing its vitality, initiated a project radically different from that of contemporaries such as Balasaraswati. Moreover, while Rukmini Devi's career path led from global experiences with dance to local ones, Balasaraswati traveled in the reverse direction: she drew from a local practice and then embarked on a global performance career.

Whereas critics hail Rukmini Devi as a pioneer, they celebrate Balasaraswati as a purist; whereas Rukmini Devi revived a tradition, Balasaraswati preserved one. Balasaraswati foregrounded this role and saw herself as safeguarding, not resuscitating or improving, an artistic legacy. She gave precedence to the dance heritage itself over any singular contribution she could make as an artist. Both her goals and her background diverged from Devi's: she sought to uphold a practice that, she argued, had already achieved perfection.[27] Nonetheless, like Devi, Balasaraswati deployed a modern discourse of creativity in her representation of bharata natyam, one that pivoted upon expressivity rather than innovative composition. She emphasized the experience and projection of interior states in performance over original authorship.

Balasaraswati shared a strategy with Rukmini Devi when she supported her decisions through an understanding of history. For Balasaraswati, however, authority lay with the devadasis and with the very practices that Devi eschewed. She identified devadasis as the rightful guardians of bharata natyam because of their direct link to the oral tradition of southern India's historical cultural center, the eighteenth- and nineteenth-century Thanjavur court. She learned dance under one mentor, Kandappa Pillai, and espoused an allegiance to the Thanjavur court lineage to which she and her guru belonged. Balasaraswati thus saw herself as responsible to the cultural inheritance of her family, community, and dance style. She defined the parameters of ideal performance practice in adherence to the protocol established by the gurusishya oral tradition. She demonstrated this allegiance to nineteenth-century dance practice by performing customary margam items deploying lyric rather than narrative modes and by retaining, as much as possible, the teaching methods of the gurukula system. In both pedagogy and performance, she struggled to retain facets of traditional protocol.

Balasaraswati, like Devi, composed kuravanji dance dramas, which her students performed, and she included compositions that previously had appeared only in music concerts in her solo repertoire.[28] She put forth these new works and performed in ensemble pieces, such as kuravanjis and Sanskrit dramas, but maintained that these were separate projects that did not and should not inform classical bharata natyam (Balasaraswati 1988: 38). Instead, she argued that the dancer's original input into the form came not through incorporating new pieces into the bharata natyam repertoire but through the expressive opportunities offered by improvisation, especially in the abhinaya aspect of conventional performance.

Balasaraswati retained the movement vocabulary, style, and repertoire of the Thanjavur court tradition in which she trained. The adavus of this style are similar in name and shape to those of the Pandanallur tradition that Rukmini Devi deployed. Although different instructional lineages feature adavus that are specific to them, the overall vocabulary and its system of classification remain consistent from one style to the next. The method of rendition, however, diverges. A Kalakshetra dancer snaps the limbs into a firmly angled position; a student of Balasaraswati eases them into a gently articulated gesture. Both styles, in keeping with conventional features of most classical Indian dance forms (Vatsyayan 1992), take the angles of the joints as a fundamental means of organizing movement. However, the Kalakshetra dancer reaches out into space, while a dancer in Balasaraswati's style retains an internal focus. Balasaraswati's students likewise give a leisurely quality to transitional movements, especially those of the hands and arms, while Devi's attention to accuracy encourages a staccato articulation of arm and head movements. Balasaraswati's emphasis on lyricism manifests it-

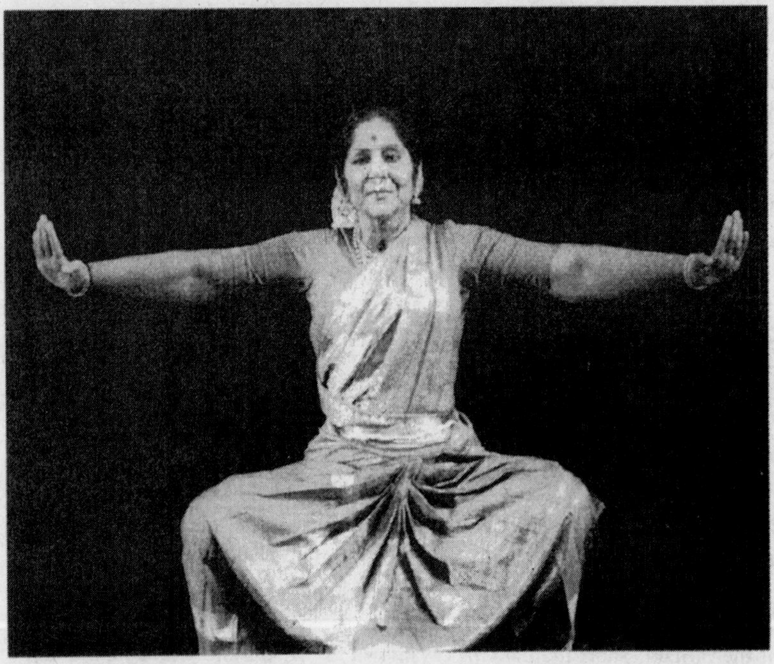

Figure 8: Balasaraswati performing an alarippu. © Jan Steward 1986.

self even in abstract phases with no dramatic content; Rukmini Devi's interest in precision appears in expressive as well as rhythmic material.

Balasaraswati drew upon the oral tradition of the Thanjavur court style in her choice of repertoire, favoring items she inherited over those of her own composition. Whereas Rukmini Devi preferred the clarity and dramatic force of multiple performers carrying consistent roles, Balasaraswati emphasized the challenges offered to the solo dancer by the lyric mode's shifting characterization. She retained the traditional poetic format, examining the emotional nuances of a specific dramatic moment rather than taking the audience through a series of events.

Balasaraswati maintained that this lyric mode and the opportunity it gave the soloist for multiple, shifting characterizations offered a unique opportunity for creative expression. She highlighted the scope for dramatic interpretation that such a format afforded the individual performer, arguing that this creativity came through adherence to traditional protocol, not in spite of it. She emphasized improvisation rather than composition, achieving renown for her inventive and evocative *sanchari* bhavas, or elaborations of the sung poetic text of a piece Such was her skill at improvisation that, according to the American ethnomusicologist Robert Brown, Balasaraswati performed the same piece fifteen times during a concert tour, yet rendered each version anew by deploying a wide range of references and poetic tropes in improvised sections (1986: 7).

Similarly, some additions to Balasaraswati's repertoire came through decisions made in improvised performance. She first performed her signature piece, *Krishna Nee Begane Baro*, as an improvisation (Raman and Ramachandran 1984a: 27). During a recital that she gave when she was fifteen years old, her mother Jayammal sang the *padam Krishna Nee Begane Baro* as a musical interlude. Balasaraswati joined her with abhinaya and improvised the rendition of the song. Over time, she refined the item and it became one of her most celebrated performance works (ibid.).[29] This process, which added a new item of choreography to her repertoire, illustrates the importance she gave to improvisation rather than preplanned devising.

Tradition, Balasaraswati argued, not only provided a dancer with scope for dramatic exploration but also offered an ideal aesthetic frame through which she and her audience could access this expressivity. The margam begins with an abstract invocation, or alarippu, moves through to the jatiswaram, a highly technical piece, and the *sabdam*, a work that juxtaposes thematic and rhythmic dance, reaching its apex in the dramatic development and rhythmic complexity of the varnam. Short dramatic pieces known as padams and *javalis* follow, and the concert concludes with the *tillana*, a dynamic, virtuoso item. Balasaraswati explained the logic for this ordering, drawing parallels between dance, temple architecture, and ritual practice (1991: 10–11). She maintained that this concert structure embodied a unique aesthetic logic without which the form no longer cohered.

Balasaraswati defended tradition by proposing an aesthetic and conceptual framework for adherence to performance conventions and validating them through reference to temple praxis. She also examined them through modern discourses of creativity, where an explicit discussion of interiority and the strategies needed to invoke it came to the fore. In performance, in her discursive representations of bharata natyam, and in her teaching, Balasaraswati emphasized the cultivation of emotional states. She maintained that the successful rendition of improvised sequences required attention to interiority. For a dancer to convey the mood of a piece effectively, Balasaraswati argued, she must develop within herself a sense of the sentiments specific to the song as well as an overall tone of devotion. This explicit discussion of the devices a performer should use to foster bhava and *bhakti*, or devotion, while drawing upon traditional South Indian aesthetics also aligned bharata natyam with a global discourse on expressivity in artistic practice, especially as articulated in dance modernism. It is not surprising, then, that Balasaraswati's emphasis on interiority gained the approval of premodern, early-modern, and modern dancers in North America.[30]

In her teaching, Balasaraswati sought to uphold traditional modes while adjusting them to new contexts. She strove to recreate the one-on-one training methods typical of the gurusishya system, whether providing instruction in her home or in a more formal environment. Although she adapted her approach to include group classes in which students practiced adavus together, she taught her most serious students both technique and repertoire in private classes. Even when teaching delimited classes in an institutional environment, Balasaraswati's teaching method was informal and flexible, introducing new material when the student appeared ready rather than when she had completed a specific set of tasks as laid out in a syllabus.

She could not, however, avoid modernizing the teaching process at the same time that she sought to preserve its tenets. She taught dance in environments different from those a traditional mentor would encounter: she gave instruction at the Madras Music Academy and subsequently held residencies at universities and arts organizations during her foreign tours. Although Balasaraswati initially taught abhinaya, encouraging her students to learn nritta with her mentor's son, Ganeshan Pillai, practical concerns, such as Pillai's ill health, pushed her to abandon this conventional division of labor. Furthermore, although she defended her community's role in the creation and maintenance of classical bharata natyam, she taught upper-caste and foreign dancers. Students from both groups pursued intensive training with her although they did not always have access to the same kind of long-term, on-site immersion that disciples benefited from in the traditional gurukula learning experience.[31]

Despite these modifications to pedagogy, Balasaraswati nonetheless privileged learning through direct practice rather than theoretical study. Although she, like Iyer and Devi, described the *Natyasastra* as the source of all classical Indian dance forms (1988: 38), she rejected the move to integrate Sanskrit aesthetic theory into dance training, arguing that understanding comes through praxis, not through textual analysis.[32] She likewise criticized an overall impetus in the dance field to evaluate bharata natyam according to the tenets of the sastras. Balasaraswati argued that bharata natyam, and sadir before it, already accommodated the principles of the Sanskrit texts and that the dance form required no modification in order to do so more effectively (1991: 12). She further maintained that regionally distinct and historically mutable "ways of life" embodied the values of canonical texts while, paradoxically, appearing to diverge from them (ibid.). Therefore, she maintained, the impetus to reform bharata natyam by associating it more closely with aesthetic theory was misguided (1984: 14).

In arguing for the value of recent historical precedent, Balasaraswati maintained that the traditional form already constituted a creative art. This premise served to cement bharata natyam's status as a theatrical, rather than ritual, practice. In addition, when she valorized the devadasi tradition, Balasaraswati explicitly acknowledged that stage performance differed from ritual service. Although she expressed religious devotion through her performance work, she rejected the impetus to "reritualize" bharata natyam, contesting the claims made by other dancers that they enhanced the dance form's spirituality when they modified performance protocol by performing obeisance to the stage and placing religious icons in the theatrical space. She insisted that dancers recognize the difference between ritual dance and the stage version of bharata natyam, urging performers to confront their new role honestly and not claim to "put the temple on the stage."[33] Her determination to acknowledge the difference between ritual and concert practice consolidated bharata natyam's position as autonomous art by emphasizing interiority over explicit display and by calling attention to, rather than masking, the function of bharata natyam as a creative performance practice in a modern, urban context.

Balasaraswati also helped to solidify the gains of the revival, paradoxically, by fighting the tide of change. The emphasis she gave to maintaining, rather than reforming, the repertoire and protocol of the Thanjavur court style gave the revival a sense of continuity. For viewers, critics, and performers, her presence in the arts as an heir to the devadasi legacy and her steadfast resolve to maintain her dance heritage indicated that despite the numerous changes wrought by the anti-nautch movement and by the revival, bharata natyam retained a connection to its past. Through her efforts, the revival operated, at least in part, as a continuation as well as a rebirth. For these reasons, dancers, critics, and spectators invoked Balasaraswati's name as a symbol of continuity throughout the twentieth century.

Balasaraswati, in contrast to Rukmini Devi, foregrounded the importance of tradition, a concept more rigid in its definition than classicism. Nonetheless, she extracted for her attention the elements of this heritage, such as interiority and expressivity, that intersected with a modern understanding of creativity. Like Devi, Balasaraswati emphasized the values rather than the form of aesthetic theory texts, although she argued that dancers' recent historical practice already accommodated such tenets and that dancers need not turn to ancient texts for guidance. Both Rukmini Devi and Balasaraswati mobilized Indian epistemologies and specific, local aesthetics as frameworks for understanding and theorizing a range of practices, including non-Indian ones (Balasaraswati 1988). Moreover, both assured that bharata natyam could travel nationally and internationally at the same time that they challenged Orientalist assumptions by locating creativity in a traditional practice. Balasaraswati extended this anti-Orientalist move when she suggested that text be understood through praxis rather than vice versa.[34] Balasaraswati argued that specificity in practice manifested the values of a universalizing textual tradition, suggesting not that practice accord itself with theory, but that only praxis-based traditions could truly realize the values of the treatises.

Balasaraswati and Rukmini Devi, despite their differing aims and choreographic projects, shared a fundamental assumption: that a bharata natyam dancer best demonstrated originality through fidelity to the past. Each located tradition in an originary moment that defined the parameters for individual contribution. Both maintained that this classical practice allowed them room to exercise creativity and imagination. Through this position, they aligned their understanding of bharata natyam's history with international discourses on originality and autonomous art while reinforcing the dance form's connection to a local and national heritage. As they had the case of tradition, they proposed different definitions of creativity, identifying it with authorship and expressivity respectively.

Each of these concerns facilitated the dancers' transactions with national and global discourses of artistic production. Rukmini Devi took inspiration from the European ballet revival of the early twentieth century, which, colored by discourses of modernism, emphasized the role of the choreographer as innovative author. Because Devi interacted with ballet and not with the emergent modern dance, and because she espoused a nationalism rooted in cultural revival, however, she located invention in the recrafting rather than the replacement of a tradition. Balasaraswati spent the first decades of her performing career in India and directly encountered a global dance context only in the 1960s, beginning with the East-West Encounter in Tokyo in 1961. When she performed in the United States for the first time, at Jacob's Pillow in 1962, it was at the request of Ted Shawn (La Meri 1985: 12); she subsequently won acclaim not only from Shawn but also from Martha Graham (Raman and Ramachandran 1984b: 26; Cowdery 1995: 5). Modern dancers found in her assertion that individual, emotional experience articulated universal themes a corroboration of their own views on artistry, which had been challenged by the subsequent generation of postmodern dancers. Likewise, Balasaraswati's foreign students found expressivity a lure because, for them, bharata natyam offered an avenue toward an interiority that the other dance forms they experienced lacked (Cowdery 1995: 51, 55).

These two legendary figures, despite their competing visions, shared the basic premise that individual expression could manifest itself in a dance that acknowledged, explicitly and in choreographic form, a debt to earlier practice. In doing so, they helped to forge a legacy through which bharata natyam articulated the concerns of both historicity and originality. Early-twentieth-century practitioners positioned these concerns in dialogue with global discourses on dance, an impulse that extended into the latter part of the century. This multifaceted ability of the dance form enabled its performers to contend with national and international demands for indicators of both authenticity and invention.

Antiquity and Creativity in Late-Twentieth-Century Choreography

Late-twentieth-century dancers who identified their work as bharata natyam, rather than as Indian contemporary dance, retained the fundamental premise put forth by Balasaraswati and Rukmini Devi: that bharata natyam best expressed originality through allegiance to tradition. These performers, like their predecessors, situated originality within classicism. They too defined tradition and classicism through specific histories that they proposed for the dance form. From the parallel, if contrasting, projects of Balasaraswati and Rukmini Devi, these performers inherited strategies for negotiating the concerns of innovation and tradition. However, subsequent generations of dancers refigured this heritage, drawing out specific components of past practice and reflecting on them in a variety of new ways.

For example, many later practitioners concurred with Balasaraswati that the solo margam repertoire afforded the individual performer the greatest scope for dramatic interpretation. Some dancers, such as Balasaraswati's senior disciple Nandini Ramani, deploy this expressivity in order to maintain their mentors' stylistic and repertory legacy. Others divide definitions of creativity, finding originality in the composition of new ensemble works while also pursuing the opportunities for dramatic rendition that solo performance provides. The 1980s and 1990s also saw an increased interest in reconstruction projects that carried out a more overt inquiry into the distant past while also providing ample opportunity for the production of new choreography. Dancers based such endeavors on, for example, the temple repertoire, Sanskrit texts, and visual iconography.

Late-twentieth-century bharata natyam retained an attention to past practice but also broadened and deepened the inquiry into history, drawing on a wider range of sources and identifying these traces of the past more explicitly in choreography. Performers made their engagement with the past more apparent than it had been previously. At the same time, however, the demand for new work also increased, especially internationally. The bharata natyam milieu of the late twentieth century also encouraged experimentation more actively than in the earlier decades.

The interest in producing works that are at once both original and classical accelerated in response to different political and economic factors from those of the early century. These include an increased attention to, in Arjun Appadurai's (1996) terms, "intentional cultural reproduction" on the part of larger and more globalized diasporic South Asian communities. Appadurai suggests that immigrants seek out emblems of cultural identity because their diasporic position requires the transmission of culture to be explicit rather than tacit. Regional and even national difference, especially for the elites of these communities, fades in relation to the threat of "Westernization." Such immigrants seek out cultural reproduction in specific practices, finding evidence in them of cultural affiliation.

Bharata natyam provides South Asian communities with a potent symbol of cultural identity because of the conjunction that revival-period dancers and promoters established between nationality, spirituality, and feminine respectability. Although some practitioners contested Devi's alterations to the form, none, other than Balasaraswati, explicitly challenged her attempt to shift the dance form to "women of good families" (Sarada 1985). Devi's standardization of pedagogy and performance established dance training as a respectable practice for young Indian women. As I discuss in more detail in chapter 3, this new reputability cemented the dance form's popularity by mobilizing an association of femininity with cultural heritage and therefore with national identity. The revival established a relationship between bharata natyam and middle-class respectability, femininity, Sanskrit traditions, and pan-Indian Hindu religious themes. As chapter 2 indicates, however, the dance form remains tied to regional as well as national identities, and it therefore operates as only a partial signifier of Indianness in non-Tamil India. The nationality of bharata natyam appears most convincing abroad, where both its disreputable traces and regional and linguistic specificities seem all but invisible. In a diasporic context, the association of bharata natyam with nationhood and respectable femininity overshadows other resonances of the dance form.[35]

The practice of bharata natyam therefore endorses an allegiance to a homeland on the part of South Asians outside of the subcontinent. For these individuals, bharata natyam expresses a set of "traditional Indian values" (Gaston 1991) that endure over time. Diasporic South Asian communities locate respectability and cultural continuity in bharata natyam. For example, Chennai-based dancers, including Nandini Ramani, Chitra Visweswaran, and Vyjayantimala Bali (personal correspondence 1999), noted that nonresident Indian communities value "traditional" elements of performances. Likewise, Gaston reports that "expatriate communities consistently place a greater emphasis on the religious or devotional elements of the dance" (1996: 318). Such groups request of both immigrant and Indian dancers overt displays of tradition, eschewing reference to the transformations the dance form underwent during the twentieth century.

This association of bharata natyam with "traditional" Indian culture has bolstered the dance form's popularity. The connection of bharata natyam to Indian, or even South Asian, identity encourages large numbers of girls to take up bharata natyam training. Although most pursue this study as a hobby, many others aim for a performance career. The diasporic demand for cultural symbols results in a proliferation of trained amateur dancers while, ironically, encouraging large numbers of young women into pursuing dance as a career.[36] This surplus, in turn, puts pressure on dancers to differentiate themselves from their peers through the authorship of original works, while the importance of bharata natyam as a cultural emblem encourages performers to demonstrate their fidelity to the past. Within South Asian communities, dancers benefit from highlighting their allegiance to tradition, but they also find that they need to distinguish themselves from amateur practitioners by illustrating their creativity.

Outside of diasporic communities, however, the situation differs. The twentieth century saw shifts first toward and then away from classicism, in public demand for Indian dance within the mainstream non–South Asian dance milieu.

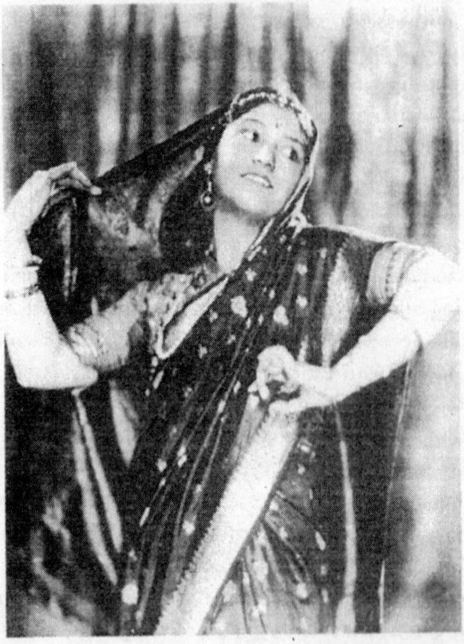

Figure 9: Ragini Devi. Courtesy of Jerome Robbins Dance Division, The New York Public Library for the Performing Arts, Astor, Lenox and Tilden Foundations.

From the 1910s to the 1940s, audiences outside of India and the South Asian diasporas attended concerts of interpretive work based on Indian themes and aesthetics, including those of La Meri, Uday Shankar, Ragini Devi, Ruth St. Denis, and Anna Pavlova. By 1935, Ragini Devi had turned to classical Indian dance. Uday Shankar returned to India, and subsequently, in the post-independence period, the popularity of his work waned, both in India and internationally. Also in 1935, Ram Gopal brought classical Indian dance to the international dance sphere. Gopal, whose concerts deployed the movement vocabulary and the repertoire of bharata natyam and other classical forms, began his international touring career during the early years of the bharata natyam revival. He achieved renown overseas with his contemporary stagings of classical choreography, selling out theaters in London's West End. These performances included margam items choreographed as duets and trios, with the pieces clustered thematically so that they formed an interlinked whole. Subsequently, Balasaraswati, embracing a more specific understanding of tradition, brought her margam-based solo concerts to prominent venues in the United States, Europe, and Asia from 1961 until the early 1980s. Thus, early-twentieth-century viewers, both in India and abroad, supported the performance of Indian-themed interpretive work, but the mid-twentieth century saw a turn away from such material and toward work that demonstrated classicism.

In the 1990s and into the twenty-first century, however, public perception came full circle, witnessing a split in international bharata natyam choreography between those works created and performed for "community" versus "mainstream" audiences. Viewers and funders situated internationally have again turned toward innovative modern and postmodern works in the South Asian dance field, seeking out choreography that intersects with Western contemporary aesthetics. Especially in North America and Britain, non–South Asian audiences, promoters, and funders favor explicit markers of experimentation in the bharata natyam–based choreography they patronize. Spectators privilege pieces that participate in a global art milieu rather than those that retain traditional aesthetics.[37]

Enduring Orientalist viewpoints alongside a lack of familiarity with choreographic codes often lead non–South Asian viewers to assume that bharata natyam choreography, no matter how recent its composition, is "ancient" and "traditional" unless its innovative moves manifest themselves explicitly. Although creativity is not restricted to choreography that demonstrates modernist or postmodern aesthetics, many international audiences require clear indicators of (Western) contemporary aesthetics before they identify a work as innovative. Some dancers argue that this kind of work receives the most funding of all South Asian–based dance material (Ramphal 2003: 32). At the same time, however, the same viewers seem to expect convincing markers of Indianness from bharata natyam–based choreographies in order to differentiate them from Western contemporary dance or Indian modern dance. Thus, in order to extend their work beyond diasporic South Asian communities, dancers based or touring abroad demonstrate both the historicity and originality of their performance projects.

In Chennai (as Madras was renamed in 1996), dancers encounter different expectations from those in cities abroad. Because Chennai played a key role in reestablishing bharata natyam, for at least some of its denizens and venue organizers, overt markers of classicism and continuity remain more important than indicators of innovation. The city's relationship to national and regional political movements extended, in a postcolonial context, an imperative to demonstrate indigeneity: that which appears too "innovative" runs the risk of looking "Western" (Menon 1998: 46; Chatterjea 2004a: 116–18). At the same time, a surplus of classical dancers and traditional performances (Coorlawala 1996: 71; Gaston 1996: 119–21; Meduri 1996: xl) encouraged dancers and spectators alike to seek out examples of new creative works. Dancers in the city found it necessary to differentiate themselves from their peers by proposing new ideas for performance works that nonetheless exhibit indicators of traditionalism.

Both inside and outside India the surfeit of trained bharata natyam dancers prompts performers to distinguish themselves from their peers by creating choreography that is original. At the same time, to remain within the sphere of classicism, dancers identify the historical basis of their work. Those who perform outside of India grapple with the contradictory demands of South Asian community and "mainstream" audiences, both of whom demand demonstrations of "authenticity" and of accessibility, but who find these elements in contrasting aspects of performance.

Late-twentieth-century dancers responded to competing demands for innovation and classicism by creating choreography that drew upon historical sources in new ways. These practitioners, like those of the revival, identified as "traditional" an adherence to the values of an overarching, originary form, which they defined in contrasting terms. Dancers expanded possibilities for innovation, however, by drawing upon a wider range of sources than their predecessors had done, located in both historical and living movement practices. A greater specificity in the inquiry into the past combined with an increased interest in creative exploration. Like revival-era dancers, late-twentieth-century performers proposed histories for the dance and suggested means for recreating the qualities of a primary form in choreography. These projects provided for new interpretations of bharata natyam's structure and content.

The Chennai-based dancer Padma Subrahmanyam maintains that her choreographic endeavors return present-day dance practice to a standardized, sastric form. While researching the *Natyasastra* for her doctorate, Subrahmanyam encountered descriptions of *karanas,* fundamental units of movement. She took the canonical status of the *Natyasastra* as an indication that the text described a germinal practice. This originary form, she argued, brought forth the regional variations that exist in the present. Based on the aesthetic theory text's division of dance forms into *marga*, or orthodox, and *desi*, characterized by regional variations,[38] Subrahmanyam maintained that classical dance should mitigate regional markers in favor of the movement priorities of the original form, as delineated in the theoretical text.

Subrahmanyam translated descriptions of karanas into movement, combining them with the basic positions and transitional movements of bharata natyam so that virtuoso turns, jumps, and leg extensions augment the adavus of the form. Her pieces resemble conventional bharata natyam choreography in that they rely on its syntax and much of its vocabulary. Her changes to the classical form came primarily through additions to rather than the replacement of its vocabulary through the inclusion of movement that, she argues, derives from the Sanskrit text.[39] She therefore suggests that the material she has created adheres to classical precedent more closely than "regional" forms such as sadir did, arguing that *bharata nritya*, the new dance form that she developed through reconstruction, revivifies an originary practice.

In her 1979 publication *Bharata's Art Then and Now*, Subrahmanyam simultaneously deconstructs claims to authenticity and replaces them with her own understanding of an essential form. She argues that any heritage must include change: "Traditions have been a continuous process. Every new element takes time to get permeated into the field and once it gets established, it joins the tide of tradition. This is how tradition itself grows" (1979: 93). Likewise, she interrogates arguments based on historical authenticity, maintaining that

> the so-called traditional concert of *Bharatanatyam* is by itself a product of the changing time. The presentation has gone through enormous changes in the past forty or fifty years. Hence, it is easy to imagine the changes that could have taken place in the last 300 years and the last 3000 years. Who could say which is original, pure and authentic. (1979: 92)

Yet, she returns to claims of historical validity when she debunks sadir's traditionalism. She maintains that the relative novelty of the form and its divergence from the hegemonic textual tradition negate the claims a dancer might make for its conservation: "The *Sadir* is itself only hardly [*sic*] 300 years old. It has its own connection as well as discrepancy from Bharata's *Natyasastra*" (1979: 92). Subrahmanyam challenges practitioners' arguments that bharata natyam's value lies in a continuous tradition that extends back to a distant past. Rather than deconstructing the notion of classicism as synonymous with venerable practices, however, she replaces one construction of history—in which bharata natyam retains authority because it is ancient—with another one in which the *Natyasastra* is canonical, and sadir, because it deviated from the tenets of the text, was not (1979: 76–77).

Like Rukmini Devi and Balasaraswati, Padma Subrahmanyam posits that creativity emerges in relation to bharata natyam's history. This past, in turn, sets the boundaries for acceptable change (Subrahmanyam 1979: 93). She follows Devi's lead when she refers to distant origins for bharata natyam and separates her choreography from the dance form's recent antecedents. However, the early-twentieth-century practitioner located in sadir artistic accomplishment compromised by the lifestyle of its practitioners; for Subrahmanyam, the movement vocabulary itself, as well as its idioms and its context, contributed to the dance form's ostensibly attenuated state. Although she expresses respect for particular devadasi dancers (1979: 91), she nonetheless maintains that sadir did not equal the dance described in the Natyasastra (88–89). Similarly, she contests the position of many of her colleagues by querying the aesthetic authority of the Thanjavur legacy, especially that of the much-valorized Thanjavur Quartet (85).

Like Rukmini Devi, Subrahmanyam proposes a history long enough that it includes change. Subrahmanyam argues against fixity within sadir itself, stating that because it has endured only three hundred years, its claim to traditionalism remains partial. Likewise, she maintains that its legacy cannot preclude transformation. Subrahmanyan, in a move parallel to Devi's, circumvents any remaining stigma on dance by evoking the unquestionably authoritative Sanskrit dramaturgical text as the primary influence on her choreographic practice. She makes a more far-reaching claim than her predecessor, however, when she indicates that she reaccesses the content and form, not just the values, of the inceptive dance practice. Although for Devi the Sanskrit texts provided inspiration, for Subrahmanyam they constitute the source of classical dance. Subrahmanyam's investigation of the distant past provides historical evidence that supports the changes she introduced to bharata natyam. This, in turn, helped to establish her singularity as a choreographer and performer and to distinguish her work from other inquiries in bharata natyam. Just as Rukmini Devi aligned her innovative ventures with the aesthetic values of the past, Subrahmanyam exercises creativity through her investigation of an earlier practice.

Vyjayantimala Bali, by contrast, foregrounds the historical legacy of the Thanjavur region. For her, traditionalism means adherence to the tenets of the oral tradition as transmitted by her mentor, Kittappa Pillai, and in her performance work she presents margam items from this stylistic lineage. Her approach parallels that of Balasaraswati in that she strives to uphold the Thanjavur tradition, as handed down by Isai Vellala practitioners, and not allow it to be diluted by hybridizing influences. Like Balasaraswati, she sees this allegiance to tradition as enabling rather than precluding personal expression.

In contrast to both of the early-twentieth-century practitioners, however, Bali emphasizes the temple tradition of nineteenth-century solo female dance. With the assistance of her guru, she reconstructed a number of items from the Thanjavur region's devadasi repertoire, basing their design on existing musical scores and on research into temple performances and rendering them in performance through the bharata natyam movement vocabulary and phraseology, which she acquired in her training.[40] Bali sees this project as one of resuscitating the source choreographies, suggesting that her original input lies not in the creation of new works but in the idea of reintroducing temple material into concert performance and the groundbreaking research that led up to the performance of these items.

In integrating ritual repertoire into the margam so that temple and court items appear alongside one another, Bali deploys elements of both Balasaraswati's and Devi's strategies. Like Balasaraswati, she associates her work with an oral tradition and connects her undertakings to the recent, rather than distant, past. She maintains that an allegiance to bharata natyam's history articulates itself best through preservation of movement vocabulary, the solo format, and a concert order based on that of the margam. She further emphasizes conservation when she describes her reconstructions as the reviving of "old and forgotten forms" (Bali, biographical sketch, promotional materials 1999).

Bali's approach also parallels that of Devi, however, when she embraces the opportunity to craft performance material from compositions that have fallen out of circulation. As Devi did with the *Kutrala Kuravanji*, Bali locates opportunities for her individual contribution to bharata natyam in the revisiting of work no longer in the current repertoire, finding creative expression not only in composition but in the research that led up to the final product. Bali's choreographic choices, like Devi's, also render the religiosity of the dance form more explicit. By reconstructing items from the temple repertoire, Bali, like Devi, supports her decisions by reritualizing bharata natyam. In drawing together the strategies of both revival-era dancers, Bali resolves tensions between innovation and allegiance to tradition, creating new material outside the margam's genre categories but supporting these choices through identifiable historical referents.

While performers such as Subrahmanyam and Bali negotiate the competing pulls of individual expression and allegiance to the past, the Toronto-based choreographer Hari Krishnan makes explicit the contrast between innovation and classicism. Rather than updating material received from his mentor or reconstructing out-of-circulation works, Krishnan selects pieces for his concerts that exhibit traits that he identifies either as "very traditional" or "very contemporary" (personal correspondence 1999). Although he strives to retain the classical aesthetics of the repertory items that he has learned from his mentor, Kittappa Pillai, he also creates and performs new compositions. He furthermore states that all of his work, by definition, expresses contemporary values because he "liv[es] in a contemporary world" (ibid.). Although he maintains that his dance "is not about extremes,"[41] his concert Solo Works (1999) juxtaposes contemporary works and margam items, drawing out their contrasts as well as their similarities.

When God Is a Customer, one of the three compositions featured in the Solo Works performance, juxtaposes bharata natyam padams and javalis with phrases of quotidian gesture or abstract expressionist, contemporary dance–derived movement. The former accompany sung poetry, while the latter occur alongside a spoken English translation of the padam text projected over the sound system. A. K. Ramanujan, Velcheru Narayana Rao, and David Shulman's (1994) translation of songs by the seventeenth-century Telugu poet-composer Ksetrayya inspired Krishnan's creation of the piece. Krishnan compiled a selection of the Ksetrayya songs and arranged the short pieces so that they fed into a linear narrative. Although the original poems, following genre conventions, explore the emotional nuances of particular dramatic instances, when strung together they form a single story that traces the actions and reactions of a particular character. In keeping with the erotic idiom of Ksetrayya's poems, Krishnan positions the pieces so that they recount the development and demise of a love affair between a courtesan and her patron, Muvvala Gopala, a form of Krishna.

The piece commences with a *mela prapti*, a musical item of the temple repertoire. As the poems begin, the lights come up slightly, and Krishnan materializes out of the shadows. Barely visible in silhouette and seated on a pedestal, he suggests, through stylized gesture, the intimate encounter between the courtesan and her god-lover. In silence, Krishnan then depicts the heroine's awakening the following day using quotidian movements like stretching his arms, throw-

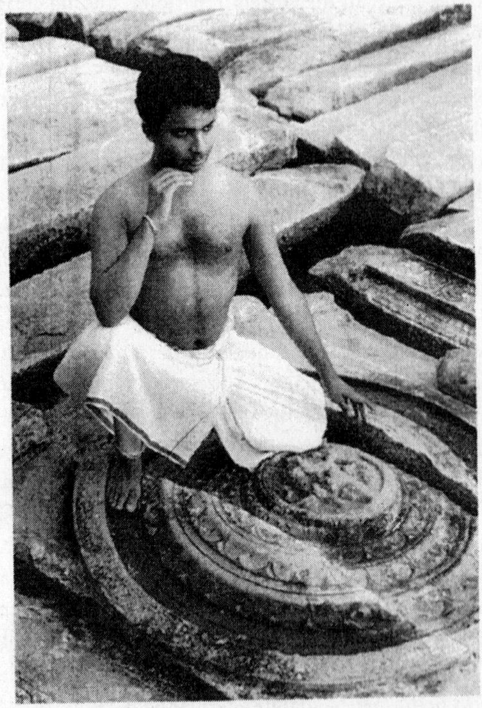

Figure 10: Hari Krishnan as nayika. Photograph by Cylla von Tiedemann.

ing back his head, and using small, delicate gestures to suggest the woman's ablutions. He holds a dignified, feminine pose, with a straight arm propped on a raised knee, during an English translation that expresses the courtesan's joy: "Today is a good day."

He stands, descends from the pedestal, and in conjunction with the sung Telugu lyrics launches a classical padam, using mudras and facial expressions to convey the mood of the song as he traverses the stage in a stately manner, walking in time to the music. In the role of the heroine, Krishnan extends his hands and draws them back, indicating a request: "Ask him to come." He then raises a hand to his forehead and extends it to the front, bowing slightly, conveying her promise to "give him a royal welcome." He develops this mood of joyous anticipation, tracing articulate hands and arms through sanchari bhavas that invoke the regal status of the absent lover. At the end of the Telugu song, Krishnan resumes a more quotidian stance as he represents the woman patiently awaiting her lover's arrival.

The piece proceeds in this manner as stylized mudras sculpt the imagery of the Telugu refrains, the tone of which Krishnan invokes through semirealistic facial expressions. During the English translation, his countenance remains neutral, and he holds a pose or performs a pantomimic gesture that conveys the sense of a single word from the line of poetry. For other sections of the English text, he employs an abstract expressionist vocabulary that suggests emotion through full-body positioning rather than through facial expression and gestures. For example, as the poetry describes the heroine's anxiety, he contracts his torso, bringing his hands to the center of his chest. He follows this sinking of the chest with a counteracting arch of the spine, led by the hands. He reaches his arms out from his center, a movement that pulls his entire torso into an open flexion and creates a vulnerable look.

As the piece winds toward its conclusion, Krishnan performs the classic bharata natyam padam *Indendu*. Dignified and disdainful, the heroine conveys her anger at the god-lover's infidelity. Krishnan's facial expressions augment the sarcastic rejoinders of the text and the mudras. He dismisses the perfidious consort with an arching sweep of his hand, his outward-facing palms signaling an unqualified rejection. Krishnan's piece, however, ends on a different note from the classical padam. He returns to the pedestal in silence, accompanied solely by instrumental music. He hovers, looking hesitantly out over the stage space, and finally retreats from its emptiness with a dropped head and slightly concave torso, suggesting that the heroine, despite her show of fury, succumbs to sorrow at her lover's departure.

The structure of *When God Is a Customer* conjoins historical source material with new choreography, exhibiting a tension between them but also suggesting their complementarity. The piece negotiates a disjuncture that early-twentieth-century practitioners encountered between narrative and lyric works as well as between the resonances of each as "innovative" and "traditional," respectively. Rather than reconstructing movement from historical sources, as Subrahmanyam does, Krishnan recontextualizes older dance material. In keeping with such a perspective, he maintains that the pieces portray the experiences of a seventeenth-century courtesan while also speaking to sentiments encountered in contemporary life: "It could be Muvvagopala of the seventeenth century or it could be John over on Fourth Street" (Hari Krishnan, personal correspondence 1999).

Krishnan's views parallel those of Balasaraswati in that he performs conventional margam items because he finds in them ample scope for dramatic expression. Like Balasaraswati, Krishnan locates universality in emotion, a commonality that endures across time and provides a link between cultures. At the same time, and in contrast to the revival-era dancer, his is an explicit project of invention. He takes an approach that is more overtly experimental than that of Rukmini Devi or of his more senior contemporaries Vyjayantimala Bali and Padma Subrahmanyam. Unlike them, Krishnan embraces experimentation for its own sake. He refers to history as a source of choreographic material but not as a standard that sets the parameters for innovation. In projecting both of these agendas in a single concert, he suggests that the two imperatives need not compete with one another or cancel each other out. He intertwines commitments to tradition and innovation without validating one through the other, indicating that the tensions between these concerns pose less of a problem for him than for his seniors.

As a Tamil dancer from Singapore who lives and presents his work in North America, Hari Krishnan inhabits a position more distant from both the devadasi tradition and the bharata natyam revival than do Chennai-based practitioners Bali and Subrahmanyam. As a man performing bharata natyam in the late twentieth and twenty-first centuries, Krishnan faces less of a stigma associated with dance than do more senior female practitioners like Subrahmanyam and Bali, who began their training and performance practice when anti-nautch criticism remained fresh in the minds of viewers. The margin between Krishnan's choreography and the censure of the anti-nautch movement that his age and gender creates enables his frank representation of the courtesan tradition. Likewise, his temporal and geographical separation from the nationalist reclamation of bharata natyam renders his position less subject to demands for authenticity, facilitating his presentation of new work. His position as a male dancer also releases him from an ostensible concordance between femininity and tradition, which accelerates demands for continuity within bharata natyam.

Krishnan, from the very position that allows him to circumvent colonial criticism and nationalist demands, grapples with the enduring affiliation of bharata natyam with femininity. For his Canadian audience, an association of South Indian solo dance with elite women intersects with a European and North American assumption that dance is a feminine practice. Although Krishnan adopts a female character, his appearance onstage, bare-chested, clad in trousers, and wearing minimal stage make-up, disrupts an association of this piece with drag performance. Similarly, when Krishnan steps out of his female, courtesan character in order to perform a more pedestrian movement, he reminds his audience of his separation from the character that he plays. His explicit foregrounding of authorship supports his position as a male practitioner of a presumably feminine pursuit. Krishnan foregrounds his role as choreographer, a position that, in both southern India and in North America, aligns more easily with masculinity than does that of dance performer. Similarly, the more abstract movements and neutral facial expressions that he adopts during the English translations universalize the piece's themes not only on a linguistic and national level but also on a gendered one. *When God Is a Customer* offsets a feminization of dance by making its originality apparent.

Performed in Canada, *When God Is a Customer* addresses an audience that requires more markers of innovation than a Chennai audience does to recognize a contemporary piece. The largely non-Indian North American audience that witnessed the Solo Works concert would tend to label most choreography of Indian origin as "traditional" and ancient unless actively encouraged to categorize it differently. Krishnan's experiments must be apparent for the majority of his viewers to find them legible, while Subrahmanyam's and Bali's projects, performed in Chennai, can introduce invention in more minute ways and still meet with viewer comprehension. In highlighting authorship rather than masking it, Krishnan addresses the expectations of a mainstream Canadian dance audience that craves evidence of originality. He therefore makes visible his global situation through a graphic juxtaposition of classicist and innovative agendas.[42]

Shobana Jeyasingh's Challenge to Tradition and Innovation

Shobana Jeyasingh, a contemporary British choreographer who creates works based in bharata natyam's movement vocabulary, also explicitly acknowledges her transnational situation. Like the other choreographers discussed here, she reflects on issues of traditionalism and innovation as they inform her work. In contrast to practitioners who define their work as classical, however, she eschews in-choreography references to historical source materials. In both her choreography and her written commentaries, she challenges neo-Orientalist and nationalist longings for "authenticity," refuting both an Anglo-British fascination with "ancient tradition" (Jeyasingh 1990) and an Indian immigrant longing for an unchanged homeland (Jeyasingh 1993: 8). While many bharata natyam practitioners debate parameters for acceptable change, Jeyasingh argues that transformation inheres in all forms, including those identified as traditional.[43]

Like Krishnan, Jeyasingh rejects the claim that she "updates" an ancient form (1995: 191). In response to critics who suggest that her work fundamentally alters an otherwise unchanged practice, she maintains that concepts of classicism and tradition define themselves not through an exact replication of their past, but through the consensus achieved among performers and viewers (Jeyasingh 1993: 6–7). She counters the suggestion that her work provides a singular challenge to a static orthodoxy by arguing that her oeuvre interrogates a constructed, not an inherently fixed, tradition.

Shobana Jeyasingh deploys a bharata natyam–based movement lexicon in order to create works within a high modernist tradition that avoids both narrative and lyric dramatic modes.[44] She uses neither the personally oriented, nuanced emotionality of Balasaraswati nor the action-oriented, dramatic crafting of Rukmini Devi. She eschews both the traditional exploration of a lyrical format and a contemporary classical investigation of linear narrative, highlighting instead such fundamentals as bodies, space, and time (personal correspondence 1999). Unlike the other choreographers discussed here, Jeyasingh mobilizes, modifies, and rearticulates the units of movement of bharata natyam without drawing on historical sources such as aesthetic theory texts, classical poetry, or images from temple sculpture and practice. She does not reconstruct out-of-circulation works, nor does she address the dance form's past in theme or narrative. She performs a reverse move to those who modify the classical form through attention to dramatic lucidity by basing her pieces on game structures, as in *Raid* (1995), or on representations of geography, as in *Making of Maps* (1991). In *Romance . . . with Footnotes* (1993), by contrast, Jeyasingh references bharata natyam by deploying the structure of a varnam, juxtaposing lyrical, contemplative sections with explosions of virtuoso rhythmic footwork (Rubidge 1996: 40). She deconstructs the conventional investigation of mood, however, replacing it with the exploration of the divergent spatial pathways formed by multiple bodies in complex groupings.

Jeyasingh retains the underlying aesthetic premises of bharata natyam, such as a grounded use of weight and the division of the body into triangular shapes rather than lines. She cites the "objective" nature of such movement priorities (Jeyasingh 1995: 193) as evidence of their suitability for use in formalist work but also seeks to "ask questions of the adavus" (personal correspondence 1999). Through these strategies, she uses bharata natyam to "creat[e] a new dance language" (1995). She describes her work as an autonomous venture, the primary relevance of which derives from her individual forays into structural and formal concerns and not from social or cultural issues (personal correspondence 1999).

Despite her rejection of overt markers of continuity, Jeyasingh, like classical choreographers, stakes her position discursively through reference to history. She discusses the same historical influences cited by other practitioners, such as the *Natyasastra*, the margam as laid down by the Thanjavur Quartet, and the bharata natyam revival, but she locates transformation within the practices of the past, deconstructing a "historicist" move to insert the "old" into the "new" (Franko 1989). She highlights evidence of change rather than continuity in each canonical moment, using history to validate experimentation rather than to set acceptable parameters for transformation. For instance, she describes the bharata natyam revival not as the rebirth of a vanishing practice but as a dynamic, self-conscious construction of tradition in the face of colonial criticism (1993: 7–8, 1995: 193). She likewise cites the Thanjavur Quartet and their standardization of the concert order but inverts the argument that their decisions hold an authoritative sway over the present moment. She suggests instead that this standardization, although now canonical, may have once inspired debate and controversy.[45] She similarly invokes the much-referenced *Natyasastra* but makes apparent the strategy implicitly mobilized by Rukmini Devi and Padma Subrahmanyam, maintaining that if bharata natyam has a two-thousand-year history, then it must have undergone radical transformations (Jeyasingh 1993: 7). Unlike Subrahmanyam, however, Jeyasingh does not replace one tradition with an older, apparently more valid one but instead insists that no practice, even the most ancient and authoritative ones, remains unchanged.

For Jeyasingh, moreover, bharata natyam's history is not only dynamic but

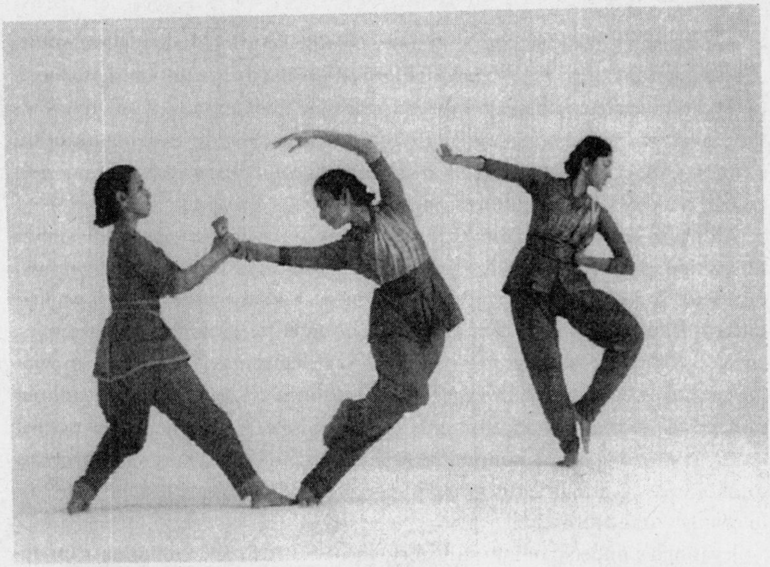

Figure 11: Shobana Jeyasingh Dance Company in *Romance . . . with Footnotes*. Photograph by Hugo Glendenning.

also hybrid. She maintains that eighteenth- and nineteenth-century choreographers negotiated, in dance material, the aesthetic preferences of the various rulers of Thanjavur (Jeyasingh 1993: 7, personal correspondence 1999), and that others, through bharata natyam, grappled with the colonial contradictions of the early twentieth century. Based on this view of history, she suggests, practitioners can also incorporate the cultural hybridity of present-day British society into choreography.

Jeyasingh identifies her work as "contemporary British dance" rather than as a cross-cultural form, reminding her viewers that, for instance, the composer she works with "lives next door . . . in Stamford Hill" (1995: 192). She makes a more radical claim when she foregrounds Britain's hybridity alongside her own: "My heritage is a mix of David Bowie, Purcell, Shelley, and Anna Pavlova and it has been mixed as subtly as a samosa has mixed itself into the English cuisine in the last ten years or so: impossible to separate" (1995: 193). In a number of her commentaries, she states that if her work reflects any kind of identity, it is a transnational, urban affiliation, not an Indian one. For instance, she describes her piece *Surface Tension* as embodying the competing but invigorating pulls between different cultural, aesthetic, and linguistic resonances of urban life (Jeyasingh, presentation, University of Surrey, Guildford, 2000).

She therefore suggests that integrating bharata natyam's movement vocabulary into British contemporary dance does not displace a fixed tradition as much as it participates in a legacy of continuous change. Jeyasingh's description of her choreography as British and contemporary allows her to circumvent the imperative within the bharata natyam sphere to celebrate tradition. Likewise, she avoids the tendency in the classical milieu to legitimize creativity by invoking historical sources. This, in turn, enables her to acknowledge multiple origins without necessarily making them manifest in choreography.

Although Jeyasingh circumvents the debates in the bharata natyam field over innovation and tradition, the set of concerns with which she contends is analogous to those faced by classical practitioners. Like the other choreographers discussed here, Jeyasingh refers to history in order to frame her choreographic choices. An understanding of the past enables change for Jeyasingh by providing not an essence, as for Devi, nor an ideal form, as for Subrahmanyam, but evidence of continuous transformation. Like Balasaraswati, she maintains that creativity has long inhered in the classical form. Unlike her revival-era predecessor, however, Jeyasingh locates creativity not in individual expressivity but also in changes to the form itself.

Jeyasingh's understanding of history, then, queries the assumption that the rigor and integrity of the bharata natyam movement vocabulary depend solely upon a relationship to the past. She also challenges the assumption that innovation is solely a twentieth-century phenomenon. By suggesting that bharata natyam–inspired choreography can incorporate modernist aesthetics on its own and that it can be innovative without integrating historical sources into choreography, Jeyasingh untangles the relationship between originality and continuity that early-twentieth-century practitioners such as Balasaraswati and Rukmini Devi established. That she does so in contradistinction to critical and spectatorial representations of her work, however, suggests the extent to which, in the bharata natyam sphere as a whole, these two imperatives remain tightly intertwined.

Jeyasingh, like the other practitioners discussed here, invokes new themes in and alongside an understanding of the past, albeit represented discursively rather than choreographically. Such historical references shed light on the classical form by indicating that even a modernist choreography rooted in bharata natyam contends with the intersecting agendas of originality and tradition and engages with an understanding of history. The understanding of history proposed by all of these artists foregrounds some sources over others, aligning bharata natyam with particular communities and therefore articulating particular politics of representation. Although, for instance, Devi's and Subrahmanyam's versions of history refer to a pan-Indian, Sanskritic legacy that frames bharata natyam and Balasaraswati and Bali emphasize a Tamil regional heritage, Jeyasingh's view of the relationship between past and present raises issues of hybridity and global interaction, deploying aspects of the past that, for her, embody Britishness and a transnational urban experience.

All of these approaches indicate a relationship between the production of history, cultural identity, and politics.[46] Bharata natyam dancers deployed their understandings of history in order to contend with the pressures placed on the dance form by colonialism, reform movements, and nationalism. The following chapters demonstrate how histories, being selections of particular elements to the exclusion of others, produce political positions. These histories, as sets of political choices, align bharata natyam with communities both "imagined" (Anderson 1991) and immediate.

2: Nation and Region

Constituting Community in South Indian Colonial Politics

Just as dancers and promoters describe bharata natyam as unproblematically ancient, viewers and performers alike also identify it as "the national dance of India." Even when not designated as the primary or originary Indian dance form, bharata natyam appears to conjure images of quintessential Indianness. The dance form articulates Hindu religious themes and recounts episodes from pan-Indian mythologies, its costuming simultaneously evokes imagery from temple sculpture and references quotidian Indian feminine attire, and its clear articulation of joints presents a set of aesthetic values that contrasts with the linearity of European forms such as ballet and ballroom dance. The intersection of bharata natyam and Indianness, like the dance form's explicit depiction of its relationship to history, however, did not evolve automatically from its past. Rather, it was produced and debated through a series of transformations that the dance form underwent in the late nineteenth and early twentieth centuries.

Like other classical Indian dance forms, bharata natyam exhibits attributes identifiable as both countrywide and specific to its area of origin, offering a productive site for the constitution of both national and regional identities. For example, the mudras that form the basis of bharata natyam's expressive language find parallels not only in pan-Indian dramaturgical texts but also in a number of regionally distinct classical dance styles. Its grounded use of weight, its creation of rhythmic phrases through footwork, and the angularity of its internal geometry (Vatsyayan 1992), although interpreted differently in various practices, connect a range of Indian dance forms. The deep bent-knee position, closed by joined heels, topped by a still torso and hips, conversely, distinguishes bharata natyam from other South Asian dance forms. For accompaniment, bharata natyam relies upon Carnatic music,[1] a style presently most visible in Chennai, but practiced across southern India. Its repertoire is multilingual, defined as much through Telugu as through Tamil and drawing upon other languages such as Malayalam, Marathi, and Kannada. Sanskrit, although primarily associated with aesthetic theory, nonetheless plays a role in bharata natyam repertoire through, for instance, the *slokas*, or short Sanskrit verses that traditionally end a concert as well as some sabdams and varnams.

National and regional affiliations appear not only in bharata natyam's form but also through its history. The bharata natyam revival emerged at a time and place in which colonial and anticolonial agitations had politicized the populace. These campaigns included nineteenth-century reform movements—which sought to align Indian social practices with the presumably universal values and standards of post-Enlightenment Europe—as well as regionalist and nationalist cultural revivals. The middle-class, Madras-based community that turned to the patronage and performance of bharata natyam during the 1930s and 1940s embraced a nationalist agenda. Revival-period dancers such as E. Krishna Iyer and Rukmini Devi located, in bharata natyam, evidence of the greatness of the Indian nation, a maneuver that, in turn, bolstered the dance practice's legitimacy as a concert art form. For the promoters of the Music Academy, bharata natyam likewise fed into a project of cultural nationalism by providing evidence of indigenous accomplishment. Therefore, as Amrit Srinivasan (1983, 1985), Avanthi Meduri (1996), and Uttara Coorlawala (1996) argue, bharata natyam's existence as a respectable, urban practice depended upon its ability to contribute to national identity.

Although bharata natyam's transformation from marginal to reputable practice hinged upon its intersection with nationalist sentiment, practitioners differed as to which communities they imagined through dance.[2] Dance practitioners and promoters diverged in their understanding of the nation's identity, its definition, and how their allegiance to it would manifest itself in choreographic practice. Performers, critics, and patrons also affiliated bharata natyam with alternate, and sometimes competing, imagined communities, especially that of the region. The region, in turn, constituted itself in divergent ways for different practitioners. For example, some performers and promoters aligned bharata natyam with the Tamil-speaking region and some with southern India more generally. In this chapter, I trace the development of a nationalist interpretation of South Indian performance through contrasting understandings of patriotism. At the same time, however, I highlight the influence on bharata natyam of another range of equally compelling discourses, those that the historian Sumathi Ramaswamy (1997) calls Tamil devotion.

The affiliation of bharata natyam with Tamil and South Indian identities either offered alternate versions of social allegiance or contributed to the dance form's status as a symbol of nationhood. When practitioners foregrounded the southern origins of the form, they aligned their projects with discourses of regional affiliation, including Tamil devotion. For these dancers, the South Indian features of the form and its history either superseded or contributed to an association of bharata natyam with Indian tradition. Balasaraswati, for example, emphasized the Tamil roots of bharata natyam and challenged an unqualified conflation of bharata natyam with the nation. By contrast, E. Krishna Iyer foregrounded patriotic sentiment but located Tamil culture at the root of bharata natyam, which, for him, then developed into a national form.

Practitioners located the political identity of dance—as national, southern Indian, or specific to the Tamil-speaking region—in their understanding of the form's past. Alongside claims to national and regional origins, performers also affiliated bharata natyam with particular castes and communities, notably Brahmans or devadasis. Similarly, they legitimized these geographico-political, class-, and caste-based links by positioning the dance in relationship to Sanskrit or Tamil literary traditions. In doing so, they expressed different opinions as to the importance of aesthetic theory—in the form of Sanskrit treatises on aesthetics and dramaturgy—to bharata natyam.[3]

Dancers thus put forth contrasting ideas of the nation and of regional affiliation, alongside caste-based belongings, linguistic origins, and literary roots, articulating these affiliations in choreographic choices and in discussions of the form. Rather than align bharata natyam with a singular political discourse, these rival nationalist and regionalist perspectives injected the dance form with the ability to represent a range of political positions. Conversely, when dancers expressed social and political affiliations in choreography, they relied upon the tenets of nationalist and regionalist movements of the late nineteenth and early twentieth centuries. Nonetheless, performers configured and represented these discourses differently in dance than did individuals in other public arenas, such as literature and governmental politics.

Despite their competing agendas and ideologies, nationalism and regionalism shared a basic aim: the defense of indigenous culture and society in the face of imperialist censure. Each set of movements contended with the investments of colonial Orientalism. Orientalism, like other colonial and precolonial discourses, legitimized imperial rule by characterizing India as in a state of decline. Colonial officials and scholars described India as incapable of equaling its former achievements and as therefore inviting domination. Paradoxically, however, the colonial characterization of India as a formerly illustrious but now attenuated civilization provided nationalists and regionalists of a variety of political persuasions with an ideological frame for crafting their counter-discourses.

The political theorist Partha Chatterjee (1986) maintains that anticolonial nationalists inverted the Orientalist problematic—arguing for Indian independence rather than for its continued subjugation—while retaining its thematics, including the contention that India's value lay in the great traditions of antiquity. This version of nationalism retained the basic ideological tenets of Orientalist thought by dividing the world into "the East" and "the West," each with its essential characteristics. Activists concurred with Orientalists that the East had a monopoly on spiritual merits and the West on material virtues, but, according to Chatterjee, they inverted the valuation given to each domain. Orientalism, although intertwined with imperialist ventures, allowed nationalists to circumvent the colonial contradictions of the present moment: if the authentic India lay in the past, then its "real" culture remained pure, distinctive, and unaltered by colonial hybridity.

Regionalists, like nationalists, challenged the colonial narrative of a civilization in decline by locating political viability in the achievements of the past. This imperative produced, in Ramaswamy's terms, a "nostalgia for civilization" (1997: 45–46). Indigenists reversed colonial charges, contending that "natives" did not need civilization imposed from without because they had always had it. The two sets of political movements differed, however, as to where this valuation lay, emphasizing particular aspects of the past and specific histories as the source of these legitimating traditions. National and regional movements therefore valorized some attributes of Indian society at the expense of others.

Ramaswamy examines one particular, highly influential version of anticolonial sentiment that she labels "metropolitan nationalism" and its underlying neo-Hindu discourses. Neo-Hinduism, according to Ramaswamy, drew from the tenets of Orientalist thought by conflating India with its spiritual accomplishments, especially those of a "pure" Hindu heritage expressed through the Sanskrit scriptural tradition (1997: 26), celebrating an ancient, elite past as the foundation of the present-day nation. Neo-Hindu activists further accepted the colonial assertion that India's most valuable traditions derived from those of "Aryan," upper-caste, largely northern Hindus (26–27). They offered a rejoinder to colonial charges of civilizational lack by locating social merit in the same cultural features that Orientalists did: Sanskrit, Brahmanism, hegemonic texts, and other forms of Brahmanical high culture. This breed of nationalism likewise deployed the colonial premise that centuries of domination had eviscerated this once-luminary civilization but emphasized the most recent, imperial invasion as the most detrimental. Neo-Hindu nationalists therefore posited a "golden age" for Indian culture in a past associated with the Sanskritic classical tradition, which predated the Moghul and British conquests. In contrast to colonial administrators, these activists maintained that India could revive its glorious institutions through a process of reconstruction and reform (Peterson 1998: 63; Gaston 1996: 346).

Neo-Hinduism also drew on the hierarchical classification of Indian races that positioned the northern "Aryan" above the southern "Dravidian" (Ramaswamy 1997: 41). Colonizers had split the Indian populace along a fundamental "racial" line, distinguishing between "Aryans," or northern, Indo-European speaking peoples, and "Dravidians," or South Indian speakers of languages such as Tamil and Telugu. Colonial linguistic surveys had found traces of Dravidian languages in North India, leading to the theory that Aryans from the north had conquered the Dravidians. Neo-Hindu nationalists deployed the colonial image of successive waves of invasion in which the noble, virile "Aryan," of Vedic and Sanskritic accomplishment, conquered the savage "Dravidian," who then retreated to South India (Ramaswamy 1997: 41). Although not all neo-Hindu nationalists disparaged Dravidian culture and tradition (Ramaswamy 1997: 27), many assimilated the colonial Orientalist disparagement of regional languages as "vernaculars" (14) and its privileging of Sanskrit, retaining a colonial racialization of language. Striving to counter a colonial narrative of Indian weakness and decadence, anticolonial activists fell back on the imperial characterization of the "refined Aryan" as emblematic of India's history of achievement.

The endurance of this racial hierarchy complicated the relationship of Tamil and of southern India to the Indian nation. As Ramaswamy (1997) argues, those invested in a Tamil identity refuted both colonial and nationalist representations of South India's ostensible cultural degradation. Early twentieth century, politically minded Tamils, whether primarily nationalist or regionalist, produced definitions of "civilization" that ran counter to both European and neo-Hindu models. Invested in a Tamil or South Indian identity, they contended with a dual Orientalism that positioned the "real" India as rooted in its past and that portrayed southern India as yet more fixed than the rest of the country. Just as nationalists did with colonial Orientalist assertions, regionalists subverted this internal Orientalism so that South India appeared as the site of enduring culture and civilization.

This chapter suggests that dancers and promoters responded to these political concerns, articulating a range of positions through colonial, national, and regionalist discourses. Central to this argument are the distinctions that Sumathi Ramaswamy draws among sets of cultural and political affiliations in late colonial and postcolonial Tamil Nadu. Ramaswamy identifies the production of Tamil identity through allegiance to language as *tamilpparru*, or Tamil devotion. The ideology of Tamil devotion and its "competing projects" (Ramaswamy 1997: 23) cut across nationalist discourses, providing indigenists with a range of political and discursive perspectives in which their dedication to Tamil Nadu supported, interrogated, or replaced fidelity to the Indian nation. Although Ramaswamy examines loyalty to the Tamil language, specifically, I suggest that her theorization of Tamil identity production extends into a broader political realm where arguments over language and social identity conjoined. Fidelity to language ran through a number of South Indian social and political movements as regionalists found allegiance less in the boundaries of the putative nation-state than in linguistic commonality. Language became further politicized after independence when the Madras Presidency was divided along linguistic lines into the Tamil-, Telugu-, Kannada-, and Malayam-speaking regions of Tamil Nadu, Andhra Pradesh, Karnataka, and Kerala.

Despite their differences from neo-Hindu nationalists, many South Indian regionalist groups preserved the idea that political viability rested upon proof of "civilization" which in turn revealed itself through "classical" traditions.[4] Civilization, for both nationalists and regionalists, operated as the benchmark of societal legitimacy. For example, in a move that Ramaswamy labels "counter-Orientalist classicism," a diverse group of Tamils, including Brahmans, Christians, upper-caste non-Brahmans, and Sri Lankans posited the antiquity and "purity" of the Tamil language as well as its distinctiveness from Sanskrit (Ramaswamy 1997: 36–38). Some of these Tamil devotees took a more "compensatory" approach, maintaining that Tamil enjoyed equality to and comparability with Sanskrit. Others favored a "contestatory" position by asserting the superiority of Tamil over Sanskrit, arguing that Sanskrit had evolved from Tamil instead of the inverse scenario put forth by Orientalists (43–44).

The group that Ramaswamy identifies as Indianist Tamil devotees mobilized their allegiance to Tamil in the interest of an explicitly political agenda, articulating linguistic fervor through and alongside demands for national sovereignty. They maintained that the interests of Tamil Nadu and the nation-state interwove and that devotion to Tamil "enable[d] participation in the Indian nation" (Ramaswamy 1997: 23). This alignment with the nation included a reconciliation with neo-Hinduism and a lack of hostility toward Sanskrit, Brahmans, and northern India (49). Indianist Tamil devotees therefore contributed to a "nation-of-nations" or unity-in-diversity patriotism that resembled that of the Indian National Congress (later the Congress Party of India). The nation-of-nations model rested on the idea that India's strength lay in its accommodation of difference. Adherents to this version of nationalism maintained that India's various local and regional practices contributed to, rather than detracted from, its identity as a sovereign state.

Dravidianism, by contrast, attacked an "imperialist" national (Indian) agenda, promoted, they claimed, by Brahmans and other elites. Dravidian activists envisioned South India as separate linguistically, racially, and politically from North India, with its apparently Sanskritic underpinnings. Dravidianists, like the neo-Hindu activists they challenged, retained a colonial racialization of language and caste. In this model, Brahmans, even those in South India, became associated with Aryans because of their historical role as priest and pundits, versed in the Sanskrit language. Dravidianists combined a suspicion toward Brahman regional allegiance (Ramaswamy 1997: 68) with a Marxist class critique, resulting in an overtly anti-Brahman position. Dravidianism, however, like other regionalist and nationalist movements, looked to history for validation, finding a legitimizing past not in Sanskrit and its traditions but in ancient Tamil literature. For these activists, works such as Sangam poetry, the *Silappadikaram* epic, and the *Tirukkural* scriptures provided evidence of the "secular" and "egalitarian" nature of Tamil culture (Ramaswamy 1997: 74).

The bharata natyam revival appears to intersect most clearly with the investments of metropolitan nationalism. Nonetheless, celebrations of Tamil heritage run through depictions of the dance form's social and cultural significance. Although few, if any, bharata natyam dancers proposed a Dravidianist view of cultural identity, most of the practitioners of the revival engaged with questions of South Indian allegiance and of a Tamil legacy. In addition, another set of intersections between colonialism, nationalism, and regionalism informed the rhetoric of the revival: the convergence between indigenist movements and agitation for social reform.

The initiators of the bharata natyam revival of the 1930s addressed a population mobilized not only by imperialism, the independence movement, and linguistic and regional affiliations, but also by nineteenth- and early twentieth-century social reform movements. Beginning in the early nineteenth century, campaigns to reform Indian society galvanized large segments of the Indian populace. Activists spoke out in favor of and against movements to change Indian social life, so that nineteenth-century Indian political campaigns focused as much on sociocultural concerns as on governmental ones. Reformers sought to alter aspects of Indian society in order to accommodate modern, European ideals of equality, while revivalists underscored the merits of "traditional," orthodox Hindu culture. Revivalists could not completely avoid colonial condemnation, so they strove to reconstruct an ancient, presumably more egalitarian Indian past (Chakravarti 1990). These agitations impelled the Indian public toward debate and political action, both by focusing on the inequities of indigenous society and by highlighting the extent to which all Indians contended with colonial values.

The anti-nautch movement belonged to a later time period than the other social reform movements but still contributed to the politicization of nineteenth- and early-twentieth-century South Indians. Although focused primarily on the dedication of women to temple service, the anti-nautch movement nonetheless brought debates over women's status in society and about the legitimacy of dance to public political discourse. The movement drew on an eclectic group of participants—British missionaries, South Indian elites, including Brahmans, and Isai Vellalas—each motivated by a different set of social and political goals.

British missionaries strove to propagate Christianity and Christian values by openly criticizing Hinduism, specifically those practices that diverged from European customs. Their participation in the anti-nautch movement was one avenue for highlighting the ills that, they claimed, Hinduism imposed on the Indian populace. The anti-nautch movement also garnered the support of urban Indian professionals. This group joined the reform movements for reasons that directly opposed the objectives of the missionaries: they sought to reform Hindu practices and align them with European post-Enlightenment values in order to validate an autonomous nation-state.

The Dravidianist "non-Brahman" activists, who by the 1920s made up the majority of anti-nautch campaigners (Srinivasan 1985: 1873) held the most complex set of views on dance and anti-dedication legislation. These individuals, like the radical regionalists among whom they ranked, pitted themselves not against the colonial powers, but against the class dominance that, they maintained, Tamil Brahmans exercised. Because they based their struggles in Marxist, rationalist thought and called for an overhaul of society, they aimed to throw off the social and political dominance of the upper castes by challenging their ritual authority and social superiority. They criticized the "superstition" of religious practice and condemned Brahmanic Hindu society for its hierarchical nature. The anti-nautch movement gave them a vehicle for leveling this critique because of the religious justification for the devadasi system and the potential for sexual and economic exploitation of devadasis by priests and other elites. For Dravidianists in the anti-nautch movement, temple dedication contributed to the subjugation of the lower castes by Brahman men.

Despite their rhetoric of class struggle, however, the Dravidianist parties consisted less of subaltern groups and more of relatively high caste non-Brahmans, including the occupational groupings associated with temple performance that came to identify themselves as Isai Vellala (Srinivasan 1985: 1869; Terada 2000: 482). In other words, the anti-nautch movement drew its ranks from the community from which devadasis were usually recruited (Srinivasan 1985: 1873). The dedication system had divided this community so that some women became devadasis while others married and joined patrilineal and patrilocal households. Devadasis controlled the economic resources of their own households, held a respected (if marginal) status in society, and were able to enter temples, while the men of their caste were not. In addition, they formed sexual liaisons with Brahman men and other elites but not with the men of their own caste group. Therefore, as Amrit Srinivasan (1985) argues, a range of motives—from sexual and economic jealousy to upward mobility—encouraged Isai Vellala men to participate in the anti-nautch movement.

According to Srinivasan, Isai Vellala men stood to benefit, in their homes and in the public sphere, from anti-nautch legislation. Through the abolishment of the devadasi system, they reversed a standard that offered devadasis a higher status than their male counterparts in the larger social milieu. And because these men were not dedicated to temple service themselves, legislation against temple service did not prevent them from continuing their roles in the performance sphere as teachers and accompanists; they retained their traditions and livelihood, while devadasis generally did not. In addition, despite their rejection of Brahman practices, the Isai Vellala community achieved greater legitimacy by adhering to mainstream (ironically, upper-caste) models of propriety (Srinivasan 1985: 1874). Conversely, their agitation contributed to the consolidation of non-Brahman caste identities through Dravidianist reform movements (Srinivasan 1985: 1873). Thus, as Srinivasan states, by the 1920s and 1930s, the anti-nautch movement "had become inextricably linked with the political aspirations of the 'Backward non-Brahmins' in Madras state" (1983: 80).

The different participants in this movement used their activism to competing ends. The missionaries strove to increase conversions to Christianity by highlighting human rights abuses in India and to contest the British government's policy of noninterference in "native" religious life. The nationalists who participated in the anti-nautch movement supported social reform in order to counter the premise that inequity in traditional Indian society justified colonial intervention. Non-Brahman regionalists, by contrast, aimed to overhaul society, modifying it along rationalist lines, through anti-ritual agitations, as well as to advance their own status. Nonetheless, each of these three groups took as fundamental the idea that social reform would strengthen political claims. Those motivated by indigenist agendas contributed to reform agitations in order to bolster national or regional movements and their accompanying claims to political sovereignty. In the process, these agitations served to politicize not only the populace, but also the discourse around dance. Thus, when a new generation of dancers turned to sadir in the 1930s, they contended with a form that had already collided with contrasting ideas of nationhood, regional identity, and equality.

The rest of this chapter traces a genealogy of the responses that bharata natyam dancers offered to questions of political and cultural identity. I investigate the different interpretations of cultural allegiance that practitioners proposed as they engaged with colonialism, nationalism, and regionalism. Although responding to similar circumstances, early-twentieth-century practitioners interpreted bharata natyam's history and aesthetic merits in divergent ways, varying in the communities that they imagined in their choreography. Thus, I suggest that bharata natyam was not simply refigured in the interest of nationalism; instead, it emerged as a platform where competing versions of identity could be staged. I examine the contrasting agendas of E. Krishna Iyer, Rukmini Devi, and Balasaraswati, as well as the institutions that supported them, in relation to the late colonial period's metropolitan nationalism and ideologies of South Indian regional pride. Despite parallels between strategies embraced by dancers, political activists, and language devotees, political claims articulated themselves differently in the dance field than in other milieus. Within the bharata natyam sphere, unlike in a wider political context, allegiances to the nation, to southern India, and to Tamil supported rather than contradicted one another.

Colonial and Anticolonial Politics in the Bharata Natyam Revival

By the time the Music Academy sponsored its first dance performance in 1931, indigenist politics in Tamil Nadu had already split into competing camps. Activists asserted Tamil linguistic and South Indian cultural identities in opposition to or in conjunction with national ones, resolving perceived tensions between them in contrasting ways. Proponents of different agendas put forth opposing claims for the preeminence of Sanskrit, Tamil, and the Dravidian language family, further associating language and regional affiliations with a range of social and political aims, as well as caste and class identities.

Music Academy officials promoted bharata natyam and Carnatic music in the interest of the nation-of-nations style of patriotism proposed by the Indian National Congress. They posited a relationship between regional and national identity that parallels the linguistic affiliations that Ramaswamy describes as Indianist Tamil devotion (1997: 61), locating national autonomy in regional allegiances and vice versa. Activist promoters asserted that regional, linguistic, and national affiliations contributed to rather than detracted from one another. Although the Music Academy aligned patriotism with regional practices, however, they also appealed to the authority of the pan-Indian traditions of Sanskrit learning as articulated through the sastras. Critics and scholars associated with the academy highlighted links between bharata natyam and Sanskrit texts, especially aesthetic theory and dramaturgical works.

While the Music Academy strove to standardize musical performance through reference to aesthetic theory (Allen 1998: 42–43), they posited a different relationship between theory and practice for dance. Scholars associated with the Music Academy maintained that the correspondence between bharata natyam, in its contemporaneous form, and sastric tenets meant that the southern Indian form expressed the values of the Sanskrit texts without requiring modification. The first issue of the *Music Academy Journal* (1930) aligned nationwide and regional aesthetics when it included an essay that demonstrated interconnections between the *Natyasastra* and bharata natyam. The Sanskritist and Music Academy officer V. Raghavan later argued that the similarities between elements of bharata natyam —including repertoire and movement vocabulary—and the theoretical categories of Sanskrit texts meant that "on the side of solo dance, as different from forms of dance-drama, the *Bharata Natya* is the national dance *par excellence*" (Raghavan 1974: 239). This argument contributed to the nationalist agenda of the organization by suggesting that bharata natyam aligned with "universal" or "country-wide" rules (Raghavan, in Peterson 1998: 41).

The appeal to Sanskrit texts had other benefits beyond sanctioning a marginal dance practice through a venerable body of aesthetic theory. Sanskrit, as an ancient lingua franca associated with elites and with a body of canonical texts ranging from religious scriptures and mythological tales to poetry and drama, offered Indian nationalists two discursive devices for opposing colonial rule. As an ancient classical language on a par with Greek and Latin, Sanskrit could challenge the colonial "civilizing mission" because it provided evidence of India's cultural refinement analogous to that used to mark the status of the West (Ramaswamy 1997: 39). In addition, as a language that appeared in Hindu liturgical and literary practice throughout the Indian subcontinent, Sanskrit provided nationalists with an already united nation on a cultural, if not necessarily political, level.

On the one hand, the Music Academy's recourse to Sanskrit as a legitimizing device paralleled the strategies of neo-Hindu metropolitan nationalists by privileging Sanskrit both as a dominant marker of aesthetic and cultural value and as a unifying force. On the other hand, these scholar-promoters used Sanskritic categories to authorize southern Indian dance practice. Music Academy officers suggested that the regional oral tradition was in itself national because it harbored common Indian artistic values. Unlike their approach to music, then, the academy's view of dance suggested that the guardians of local traditions did not need to modify their practices in order to align them more closely with the tenets of Sanskrit texts.

The academy's position suggested that regionally based forms such as bharata natyam, crafted through oral tradition over the centuries, preserved an overarching set of aesthetics shared on a national level. The approach of the Music Academy thus accords with that of the language proponents Ramaswamy calls compensatory classicists, who validated Tamil language and literature by demonstrating their equality with Sanskrit. Since compensatory classicism harmonized Sanskritic and Tamil traditions and avoided the anti-Brahman rhetoric of other regionalist movements (Ramaswamy 1997: 43), it was particularly well suited to the cultural revivalism of these largely Brahman, middle-class arts promoters.

Accordingly, members of the Music Academy, notably the dancer, promoter, and critic E. Krishna Iyer, proposed a history for bharata natyam in which national and regional roots for the form intertwined. As I suggested in the preceding chapter, bharata natyam practitioners located historical continuity in contrasting elements of dance performance. These histories, in turn, by highlighting some influences on the form over others, aligned the practice with different communities and invoked particular politics of representation. Read alongside his performance and promotional activities, E. Krishna Iyer's monograph draws together southern Indian and pan-Indian Sanskritic traditions. Iyer argued, for instance, that the Tamil and Sanskrit literary works of two millennia ago describe an almost identical dance form (1957: 11). He maintained that texts such as the *Natyasastra* referred to a dance practice with southern Indian origins that by the time of the treatise's composition had spread throughout India. According to Iyer, once Sanskrit authors standardized this dance form, it returned to the Tamil-speaking region, where its custodians safeguarded it from waves of invaders and their hybridizing influence, thereby upholding the values of an orthodox, pan-Indian tradition (23). Bharata natyam, he argued, simultaneously retained features of the national tradition and its distinctively Tamil qualities (18).

Iyer's project thus integrated Tamil classicism with Indian nationalism, representing bharata natyam as a product of a South Indian heritage that Sanskrit aesthetic theory and dramaturgy brought to full fruition. Especially when viewed in relation to Iyer's own performance of items inherited from the devadasi tradition, with pieces in Tamil and Telugu, this view of history conjoins regionalist and nationalist sentiment. It locates roots for a nationwide, Sanskrit theoretical tradition in southern Indian praxis. In performance and promotion, Iyer valorized South Indian aesthetics as they found form in the devadasi legacy, yet he maintained that these features supported, rather than detracted from, its nationality. Iyer did not simply claim the parity of Sanskritic and Tamil influences on bharata natyam, however, nor did he validate bharata natyam only by demonstrating its parallels to the tenets of Sanskrit aesthetic theory texts. Instead, he argued that the southern practice exceeded the antiquity of Sanskritic models. For him, the Tamil practice was the basis of that which the treatises described. This paralleled a more general claim that Tamil culture undergirded what was later identified as Aryan and Sanskritic.[5]

Iyer, like the Congress Party, which sponsored the Music Academy's first meeting, posited a determinative relationship between regionalism and nationality. However, Iyer did not share the Congress Party's benign attitude toward other regionally marked traditions; he compared other contemporaneous dance forms of India unfavorably with the Tamil tradition, claiming that they had emerged out of "regional, folk" practices (1957: 27). A potentially more ecumenical nation-of-nations model also runs aground on the religious biases of Iyer's tract. When he argued that bharata natyam remained true to Indian classicism, he contrasted it with the products of the Moghul courts, such as the North Indian classical dance form kathak. His claim for bharata natyam's superiority correlates Indian heritage with Hinduism.

Nonetheless, Iyer's integration of Sanskrit theory and recent historical practice is notable for the contrast it forms to the position taken by other revival and post-revival dancers. Unlike Rukmini Devi, for instance, who saw the *Natyasastra* as the source of classical dance, Iyer represented the aesthetic theory text as descriptive not generative (1957: 12). Although he approved of attempts to coordinate contemporaneous practice with the tenets of aesthetic theory (43), he suggested that bharata natyam extended a Tamil legacy that had already contributed to a shared, national tradition. By contrast, for Devi and even more for post-revival performers such as Subrahmanyam, Sanskrit theory provided the source for a variety of regional traditions.

Despite his emphasis on bharata natyam's oral tradition, E. Krishna Iyer conceded that the dance form required some modification in order to fully represent cultural accomplishment. In performance practice Iyer attempted to purify bharata natyam by ridding it of its ostensibly excessive eroticism and jocularity. His understanding of the merits of dance drew upon the values of the nineteenth- and twentieth-century middle classes that formed the support base for metropolitan nationalism. Here his project, despite its regionalist overtones, dovetailed with the more explicitly nationalist agenda of Rukmini Devi.

In contrast to Iyer's position, nationalist and regionalist discourse in bharata natyam divided in the agendas of Rukmini Devi and Balasaraswati. Although these two practitioners constructed their notions of originality and tradition around similar, if inverted, frameworks, they diverged in their understanding of bharata natyam's cultural and geographical origins, its rightful affiliations, and the necessity of reform to dance praxis. Rukmini Devi entered the field of dance with the imperative of spiritualizing the dance so that it could better express the glories of Indian culture (Devi n.d.b: 22). She felt that, in order to accomplish this, she needed to transfer the dance form to "family women" and to align it with the values of an ancient, pan-Indian Sanskrit tradition. Balasaraswati, by contrast, maintained that the dance form was perfect as it was and that it required no purification. She located its merits in the Tamil tradition and more specifically in the devadasi heritage associated with the Thanjavur court. She emphasized Tamil and Telugu items of repertoire and celebrated their tradition of sringara bhakti.

The two practitioners thus claimed different imagined communities for bharata natyam: the bulk of Rukmini Devi's comments refer to Indian tradition, while Balasaraswati's invoke a Tamil legacy. Between these two figures, constructions of history and authority divided further into a set of supporting categories that correlated with the larger-scale political debates of the time. Rukmini Devi predicated her nationalist vision of bharata natyam upon the intervention of respectable practitioners, a (re-)introduction of Sanskritic aesthetics, and a reform of indigenous practice. Her project intersected with a "neo-Hindu" spiritualization of national identity (Peterson 1998: 63). Balasaraswati highlighted South Indian origins for the dance practice and maintained that devadasi practitioners had safeguarded this tradition, locating the form's origins in the courts and temples of the Tamil-speaking region. Her view does not correspond as easily as Rukmini Devi's with broader political discourses because she did not subscribe to an explicit activist position. It does, however, bear the traces of, in Ramaswamy's terms, Tamil classicism, which aligned Tamil with European and Sanskritic definitions of civilization.

These two approaches cleaved what Iyer would intertwine, so that the dance form expressed a contemporaneous contest between national and regional identifications. Yet within each practitioner's construction of history and classicism, and especially within choreographic practice, elements of the opposite discourse appeared. Rukmini Devi's reformed, spiritualized choreography drew upon regional elements. Balasaraswati's allegiance to Tamil supported rather than detracted from bharata natyam's national associations.

Like E. Krishna Iyer, Rukmini Devi contributed to the discursive position of the institution with which she affiliated her dance work. The Theosophical Society, although also a cultural organization that conducted its activities with nationalist aims in mind, proposed a different understanding of the emergent nation and its arts from that of the Music Academy. The society sought to revivify a nationwide, modernized, rationalized version of Sanskritic culture (Ramaswamy 1997: 27) rather than promote nationalism through a variety of regional cultures.

The Theosophical Society contributed to the neo-Hindu move to spiritualize national identity, striving to coordinate contemporary social practice more closely with that of the past, especially as articulated through the Sanskrit sastras (Srinivasan 1983: 92). Theosophists, as neo-Hindu nationalists, thus struggled against colonialism while absorbing some of its criticism of living practices and its valuation of elite, Sanskritic attributes of India's past.

Along with the nationalist activists of the Theosophical Society, Rukmini Devi sought to reaccess the values of the past—exemplified by the Sanskritic tradition—through present-day practice. Devi entered the dance field with the imperative of purifying bharata natyam so that it could better express these merits of Indian culture, aiming to revise the form according to the tenets of a venerable, nationwide, Sanskrit tradition. She foregrounded a distant past in which a pan-Indian dance tradition enjoyed a high status and used this history as the basis of her refiguration of bharata natyam. She maintained that dancers could restore ancient India's former glories through the reform of tradition and the revival of the tenets of Sanskrit drama and aesthetic theory texts.[6]

If Iyer identified bharata natyam as a practice that demonstrated Tamil Nadu's ability to harbor Sanskritic traditions while retaining regional distinctiveness, Rukmini Devi made a more straightforward claim, describing bharata natyam as the national dance of India. She envisioned bharata natyam as an entity that undergirded Indian practices, stating that it expressed "the very essence of India itself" (in Coorlawala 1996: 70) and that "Bharata Natya is the root and origin of all dance in India" (Devi n.d.b: 22). She described the dance form as a primordially and quintessentially national practice, arguing that it correlated with the *Natyasastra*'s description of solo female dance and therefore that it predated other styles (in Coorlawala 1996: 69). Like the Music Academy officers, Rukmini Devi affiliated bharata natyam with the nation. However, in contrast to Raghavan, who viewed bharata natyam as an ideal dance practice *for* the nation, and Iyer, who identified an ancient version of bharata natyam as *the source of* a national dance, Devi maintained that bharata natyam was an essence, a quality shared by all Indian dance: "Essentially all real dancing is Bharata Natya" (Devi n.d.b: 22). She defined bharata natyam neither as a style nor as a tradition, but as a trait, a common quality, which in turn contributed to and undergirded all classical Indian dance. She did not explicitly counter regionalist interpretations of the dance form, but rather privileged national associations over other affiliations.[7]

Nationalist sentiment found expression not only in Rukmini Devi's understanding of history but also in her pedagogy. In institutionalizing bharata natyam training, Devi combined a modern concern with standardized, uniform teaching methods with the incorporation into dance instruction of traditional high-caste practices such as vegetarianism, early-morning prayer, and the recitation of Sanskrit verses (Srinivasan 1983: 93), linking dance training to the theosophist goal of creating a rational, contemporaneous version of Sanskritic culture (Ramaswamy 1997: 27). By infusing dance pedagogy with Sanskrit theory, Rukmini Devi aligned dance with a precolonial lingua franca, emphasizing national, rather than regional, roots for classical dance training and practice. Because Sanskrit met colonial Orientalist and nationalist standards of "classicism" and "civilization," it sanctioned bharata natyam as a respectable practice and as a symbol of a sovereign state. Sanskrit's association with caste and class identity also reinforced its nationality by referencing not only the pundits of the *agraharas*, or Sanskrit-speaking villages, but also the urban middle classes who populated the metropolitan nationalist movement.

Rukmini Devi's standardization rendered bharata natyam national on a practical level as well. By providing systematized training, Kalakshetra validated dance practice for middle-class Indians from a variety of regions. Kalakshetra also offered formal education alongside dance study and provided funding to students who required it, making it possible for young dancers to leave their immediate environment by providing the assurance that they would not compromise their education and would have some level of financial security.[8] As Coorlawala points out (1996: 67), the incorporation of Sanskrit provided not only an ideological link to nationhood but also a pragmatic one. Sanskrit, as a root of North Indian languages and an influence on South Indian ones, provided linguistic commonality for an otherwise polyglot group of students. So, too, did the use of English, India's modern de facto (albeit elite) lingua franca, as a medium of instruction. Devi's goal of "separat[ing] [her] work from the traditional dance teachers" (in Sarada 1985: 50), although not inherently nationalist, moved pedagogy away from immediate communities and opened bharata natyam up to dancers who had no local or regional links to it. Her syllabus system also encouraged bharata natyam to spread nationally. By establishing regulated, explicit methods of instruction, Rukmini Devi gave her students the means of imparting a Kalakshetra education to other dancers who had no physical proximity to the Madras institution.

The motifs that Rukmini Devi (re-)introduced to the bharata natyam repertoire also contributed to a unified image of national identity. Rukmini Devi sought out themes and compositional devices that audiences on a national level could find accessible. On the one hand, Devi choreographed works in "regional" languages, such as Tamil, Telugu, and Bengali, as well as in Sanskrit (Sundari, in Sarada 1985: 224), a strategy that, as Indira Viswanathan Peterson notes, constitutes a unity-in-diversity strategy: through them, Devi was able to draw together "a variety of languages and subcultures" (1998: 64). Devi also developed dances based on the lives of female poet-saints, including the South Indian Andal and North Indian Mira, whose work forms part of the canons of their respective regional languages as much as of a nationwide body of literature. This approach aligned her choreography with a nation-of-nations patriotism.

On the other hand, Rukmini Devi's dance dramas favored pan-Indian (Hindu) stories over local ones, a decision that aligned more with the neo-Hindu search for common national ground than the nation-of-nations celebration of difference. Although conventional items such as varnams, padams, and javalis invoke episodes from pan-Indian epics and mythologies primarily as tropes and as metaphor, Rukmini Devi's dance dramas foregrounded these tales as their central narratives. Unlike margam items that praised local kings and celebrated regional incarnations of Hindu gods, Devi's ensemble works recounted episodes derived from the Sanskrit Puranas, the Ramayana and Mahabharata epics, and from Sanskrit dramas, including narratives that appeared across Indian literatures and cultures, in addition to the more local kuravanjis.

Many of these dance dramas emphasized the heroic exploits of omnipotent gods and philosopher-kings, supplanting the intimate sringara bhakti of varnams and padams with a more direct celebration of the actions of eminent figures. These characters, contrasting with both the flawed, complex nobles and deities of the epics and the playful, fickle, and philandering gods of bhakti poems, allowed Devi to reinscribe Indian culture as spiritual, morally upstanding, and noble. By focusing on religious values and courageous actions, rather than on emotional states, Rukmini Devi's choreography dovetailed with a neo-Hindu nationalist image of a heroic and philosophical Aryan tradition. As such, her dance dramas contributed to a more general spiritualization of national identity.

Rukmini Devi introduced ascetic heroes not only through dance dramas but also through new items that she incorporated into the solo repertoire. Several of these items celebrated Siva in his form as Nataraja, or the ascetic dancing lord. As Matthew Allen suggests, Nataraja did not frequently feature in the devadasi repertoire, whose poets preferred the more human, amorous, and mischievous Murugan and Krishna for their sringara bhakti renditions (1997: 76). Devi introduced choreographic items that portrayed Nataraja's vigorous dance and his austerity in order to circumvent the negative associations that, she felt, accompanied the more erotic pieces of repertoire (82).

Siva Nataraja provided bharata natyam with a virile but austere icon. This conflation of spiritual detachment with masculine power bolstered a transnational, neo-Hindu nationalism as evoked by such figures as Swami Vivekananda. As Parama Roy argues, Vivekananda provided Indian nationalism with a means of simultaneously commending the world-denying traditions of India and countering the colonial feminization of India and Indian men (1998: 107). By linking the traits of manly vigor with asceticism, Nataraja, although represented by women in dance, could likewise "remake" India as dynamic and vigorous (Roy 1998), thereby inverting a colonial gendering of nationhood. The powerful dancing god, despite his possible southern origins, echoes the colonial characterization of the dynamic, philosophical Aryan tradition but reverses an Orientalist claim by staging these traits as persisting into the present.[9]

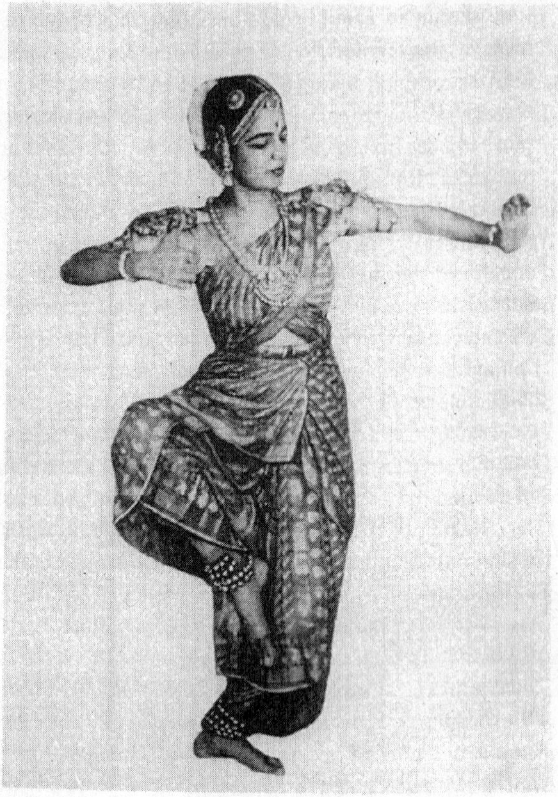

Figure 12: Rukmini Devi performing the vigorous dance associated with Siva Nataraja. Courtesy of Jerome Robbins Dance Division, The New York Public Library for the Performing Arts, Astor, Lenox and Tilden Foundations.

Despite her emphasis on Sanskrit aesthetic theory, pan-Indian narratives, and neo-Hindu icons, Rukmini Devi retained sadir's fundamental choreographic elements. Rather than reconstruct a form that embodied only common, national features in its units of movement, Devi revised the dance practice based on the Pandanallur style's vocabulary, phraseology, and repertoire. Although Devi's student S. Sarada, a Sanskritist, reconstructed phrases from the medieval Sanskrit text *Abhinaya Darpana* and integrated them into Kalakshetra training (Sarada 1985: 21), these were few in number, and, more important, they supplemented rather than supplanted the adavus as the basic units of movement for the Kalakshetra system. Sarada describes her reconstruction work as "correlating and approximating" the reconstructed movements with the "traditional usage of postures etc. in the traditional dancing of Bharata Natya" (21).

Thus, as Amrit Srinivasan (1983, 1985) argues, although Rukmini Devi overhauled bharata natyam through reference to a Sanskritic legacy, she also relied upon sadir, the very tradition that she eschewed discursively. Sadir displayed some elements shared by other regional dance forms and also incorporated features specific to Tamil Nadu—including the language of its poetic texts, movement vocabulary, and the idioms used for dramatic expression—which Rukmini Devi legitimized, rather than eradicated, through reference to Sanskrit texts. Devi used pan-Indian theoretical works and narratives—symbols of bharata natyam's enduring aesthetic and spiritual values—to frame, rather than to replace, regionally marked elements of performance. Devi thus avoided the neo-Hindu disparagement of "Dravidian" culture. Her approach aligned her project with, in Ramaswamy's terms, compensatory classicism as well as with metropolitan nationalism. On the one hand, Devi identified bharata natyam as a trait that found validation in ancient texts and that ran through a number of dance practices; she thus accorded her project discursively with neo-Hindu projects of reconstruction and standardization through reference to Sanskrit treatises. On the other hand, she relied choreographically on the very markers of regional difference she avoided in her discussions of history. When Rukmini Devi used a South Indian tradition as the basis for a nationalist interpretation of dance practice and legitimized an identifiably Tamil dance form through reference to Sanskrit aesthetic theory, she aligned her project with the compensatory classicist gestures of her predecessor, E. Krishna Iyer.

This strategy allowed Rukmini Devi to subvert colonial Orientalism. Like the imperialist discourse that preceded it, Devi's project subsumed a multiplicity of practices into a singular, originary, and hegemonic tradition and privileged an elite, Sanskritic, and textually based version of "Indian culture." Nonetheless, it also challenged the Orientalist paradigm by shifting the relationship between knower and knowledge source. In the classic Orientalist example, the information itself was Indian while those who interpreted it were European (usually German or English) men in positions of governmental or other official power. The framework for interpretation was also European, with Indian texts, philosophies, or practices explained through Western epistemologies. Devi reversed this paradigm not only because she was Indian and female, but also because she reconstructed her "ur-dance" through a theoretical frame derived from Indian epistemologies and, ultimately, from practice rather than from text. Her project was nationalist in both substance and structure.

Balasaraswati, in contrast, traced a history that highlighted bharata natyam's regional roots. Balasaraswati, unlike Iyer and Devi, did not enter the dance field through involvement with a specific political movement. However, she shared a strategy with her contemporaries when she contributed to discussions over bharata natyam's cultural origins, defending her aesthetic choices through reference to history. As indicated in chapter 1, Balasaraswati located authority in bharata natyam in gurusishya relationships that extended back to the nineteenth-century Thanjavur court. She likewise identified bharata natyam's roots as southern Indian, locating the form's origins in devadasi practice as well as in Tamil texts and the South Indian religious heritage. Through this emphasis on an oral tradition, she defended her community's practices against an impulse she saw as appropriative; at the same time, she also posited regional and local origins for the dance through reference to the recent historical past. Instead of seeking out commonalities among Indian classical forms, as did Iyer and Devi, she rooted bharata natyam in a continuous tradition of South Indian dance, music, and literature. In performance, she favored Tamil and Telugu items of repertoire and celebrated their tradition of sringara bhakti. She privileged the maintenance of this oral tradition over the reconstruction of material from Sanskrit aesthetic theory (1991: 12), defending the devadasi heritage against calls for the reform of the structure and content of performances (in Raman and Ramachandran 1984a: 30).

The history that Balasaraswati described consisted of a Tamil tradition that abided with devadasi practitioners who, in turn, upheld the aesthetic value of sringara bhakti. Authority, for her, lay within the devadasi community: she maintained that devadasis preserved a crucial link between a rich, emotional bhakti and sringara (in Raman and Ramachandran 1984b: 30). She furthermore argued that erotic sentiment contributed to a specifically South Indian dance history: "*shringara* [*sic*] . . . was pre-eminent in the Tamil dance tradition right from the beginning" (Balasaraswati 1975: 2). She claimed that Tamil, which was exceptionally well suited to the conveyance of emotional themes, particularly through powerful erotic idioms, also operated as a form of devotion: "As far as I know, Bharata Natyam is a form of *bhakti*; Tamil is also nothing but *bhakti*. I believe, therefore, that Tamil and bhakti are part of the same tradition" (1975: 1). Tamil, for Balasaraswati a language divine and classical, had the unique ability to align devotion and eroticism.[10]

In contrast to Rukmini Devi, who gave priority to the dramatic clarity of the linear narrative format, Balasaraswati preferred the emotion-driven lyric mode of bhakti poetry (1991: 6). Some of these pieces address the god-lover directly, a strategy common to devotional literature in Tamil and in other languages. Other sringara bhakti pieces, as Matthew Allen argues, exploit a device inherent to Tamil literature: a "tripartite structure" in which the heroine tells a female friend or messenger of her affection and anxiety and enlists her companion's help in retrieving her lover (1997: 75–76). This "rhetorical scheme" has appeared in Tamil literature since the Sangam period (Allen 1997: 76). Balasaraswati's decision to retain this literary device signals not only a preservationist agenda generally but also an allegiance to the conventions of Tamil literature.

An affiliation with characteristically regional aesthetics also reveals itself in Balasaraswati's celebration of the characters that Rukmini Devi held at a distance: the amorous, playful god-lovers Murugan and Krishna. This choice supports the priority Balasaraswati gave to sringara bhakti, for these worldly gods contrast with more austere deities such as Siva Nataraja and Rama (Allen 1997: 77). Balasaraswati's emphasis on the erotic idiom continued a historical appreciation for these gods as "romantic leads" that the plethora of classical songs about

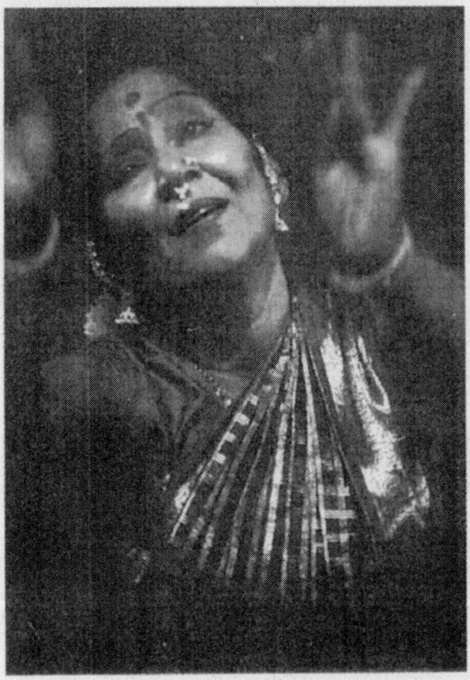

Figure 13: Balasaraswati's sringara bhakti. © Jan Steward 1986.

them demonstrates (75–76). Of the two, Murugan is the more indigenous god in that he descended from a pre-Hindu Tamil deity whom Hindus later incorporated into their pantheon. As Matthew Allen points out, in Tamil Nadu, Murugan figures as a romantic, lively, yet frequently neglectful and philandering lover, in a direct parallel to Krishna's depiction in bhakti songs in Telugu and North Indian languages (1997: 76).[11] Balasaraswati, although emphasizing the Tamil tradition and performing Tamil padams, preferred Telugu Krishna poems to Tamil Murugan songs. Through these interlinked choices, she gave primary discursive attention to Tamil but interwove Tamil into a more general South Indian cultural identity.

Despite the emphasis that Balasaraswati gave to oral tradition, she, like her contemporaries, also ascribed importance to ancient texts. She drew information on historical dance practice from some of the same sources Iyer had: the Tamil epics *Silappadikaram* and *Manimekalai*. Moreover, she cited the Tamil poet-saints in her history of sringara bhakti, arguing that these Tamil poems fed into devotionalist literary developments in other languages (Balasaraswati 1975: 2). In contrast to Iyer, however, Balasaraswati celebrated the Tamil tradition in itself rather than as the source of a nationwide tradition.

Balasaraswati shared Rukmini Devi's attention to the *Natyasastra* as the source of classical Indian dance forms (1988: 38), and like Devi she treated the *Natyasastra* not as a handbook for choreography but as evidence of the dance's origins. Balasaraswati's premise, in this sense, concurred with Devi's: she maintained that contemporaneous dance styles best honored the practices of antiquity by expressing their values, not by replicating their form. Although Balasaraswati agreed with her colleague in the revival as to the essential value of the authoritative texts, she remained critical of attempts to reform bharata natyam through reference to aesthetic theory (1984: 14).

Balasaraswati did not conflate bharata natyam with other Indian forms but maintained that regionally distinct and historically mutable "ways of life" embodied the values of canonical texts while, paradoxically, appearing to diverge from them (1991: 12).[12] Therefore, for her, local and regional traditions could express national and, indeed, universal values through their own distinctive elements, rather than in spite of them.

Balasaraswati did not reject outright the increasingly persuasive association of bharata natyam with national identity. She recognized an overarching category of Indianness, which, she maintained, encompassed a range of regionally diverse forms. She further suggested that these genres aligned themselves with pan-Indian, hegemonic practices such as yoga, Upanishadic thought, and Sanskrit theory (1984: 12). She supplemented, rather than countered, a pan-Indian cultural legacy through reference to local and regional traditions. By celebrating the Tamil legacy and the devadasi inheritance, Balasaraswati integrated the South Indian practice into a potentially national tradition. Balasaraswati's discursive and choreographic strategies correlated her position with the largely elite compensatory classicists who equated Tamil with Sanskrit, rather than suggesting that the South Indian language superseded the pan-Indian classical one (Ramaswamy 1997: 43). This approach allowed her performances to find favor both with the Music Academy and their investment in a nation of nations cultivated through South Indian practices, and with the Tamil Isai Sangam (Tamil Music Organization), which celebrated a southern Indian heritage by promoting music in the Tamil language.

At the same time, Balasaraswati's perspective did not fit easily with the largely elite nationalism of the Music Academy. She critiqued attempts to reform bharata natyam in caste- and class-based terms. Despite the close professional relationship she had with Brahman scholars, promoters, and students, she conflated reformism with caste identity when she labeled "the style of Bharatanatyam emphasizing bhakti over sringara . . . as 'brahminized' dance" (Raman and Ramachandran 1984b: 30). This challenge to reformist practices, issued along caste lines, threatened to rupture the reconciliations between nation and region, text and practice, and Sanskrit and Tamil that she proposed in her understanding of history and her choreographic decisions. Her valorization of a devadasi legacy, as the source of a Tamil tradition, paralleled the rhetoric of contestatory classicists by foregrounding a non-Brahman identity and arguing that Tamil language and culture depended on such non-elite communities for their continuance.

However, radical regionalists, especially those associated with the Dravidianist movements, had rejected sadir and the devadasi system that supported it. In doing so, they distanced themselves from the reformulation of bharata natyam (Srinivasan 1983: 91). Balasaraswati's position was therefore fraught and anomalous. She faced a changing dance milieu where the refiguration of bharata natyam as upper caste and middle class facilitated its respectability. At the same time, much of the Isai Vellala community had rejected devadasi dance. Balasaraswati was the sole representative of the devadasi tradition remaining in the public eye, and she defended bharata natyam as a devadasi domain. Yet she relied upon the support of the largely upper-caste Music Academy as well as on an international dance milieu.

Balasaraswati resolved this dilemma by deploying the notion of universality. In several of her commentaries, she referenced the universal function of dance (1991: 23), positing that all art, everywhere, fulfills spiritual ends (1988: 37, 1991: 9). Like Devi, she deployed an idea of spirituality, in addition to religiosity, abstracting bharata natyam from a relationship to only its immediate context. For Balasaraswati, however, this higher function came through emotionality and interiority, aspects that provided bharata natyam with regional, national, and global affiliations (1991: 23). Through this reference to universalism, Balasaraswati could bridge the gap between her valorization of the devadasi community and the realities of her instructional and patronage situation. This maneuver partially defused the tensions between her celebration of the devadasi legacy and her performing for and teaching Brahmans, non-Tamils, and non-Indians.

Balasaraswati's recourse to universalism suggested an international positioning for a practice with local and regional roots. It allowed her partially to circumvent issues of belonging while retaining the class- and caste-based affiliations that underpinned her traditionalist perspective. It also enabled her to teach Brahmans and foreigners and to accept the support of their institutions without compromising the heritage she valued. Her representation of the form provided an alternative reconciliation of the tensions between local, regional, and national traditions to the resolutions suggested by activists and Tamil devotees.

E. Krishna Iyer, Rukmini Devi, and Balasaraswati all contended with the intersection between bharata natyam and the politics of the emergent nation-state. However, each proposed a contrasting image of Indianness, finding national identity in different histories, practices, communities, and languages. The three also differed from one another in the relationship they posited between the nation, the Tamil-speaking region, and South India more generally, drawing upon divergent strands of contemporaneous and historical Tamil regionalist discourses. However, none of them simply capitulated to the claims made by activists. Bharata natyam was not repositioned through the revival as a vehicle of a unitary nationalism, nor was it refigured solely along the lines of linguistic and regional allegiances. Instead, through dance, the revival's practitioners posited distinct solutions to questions of social and political identity, resisting as well as deploying the dominant discourses of their time.

Nation and Region Refigured in Late-Twentieth-Century Choreography

The competing definitions of social and political affiliation with which revival-era dancers grappled had diverged further by the late twentieth century. On a governmental level, Tamil allegiance apparently prevailed over Indianism: the regionalist Dravida Munnetra Kalakam, or Dravidian Progress Association (DMK), defeated Congress in 1967 and has stayed in power since. As Ramaswamy points out, however, rhetorically and in terms of policy, Dravidianists softened their position on India by the 1970s (1997: 63) and ultimately integrated their loyalty to Tamil into a national allegiance (77). At the same time, traces of radical Dravidianist discourse still circulate in Tamil Nadu, and class and caste critiques continue to undergird some interpretations of regional identity. In addition, separatist versions of cultural identity came to the fore of political and popular discourse of the late twentieth century, albeit less in Tamil Nadu than elsewhere in South Asia. These ranged from the religious fundamentalism and regional chauvinism of Shiv Sena to the Khalistan agitations for a Sikh state in northwestern India and the separatist Tamil Eelam movement in Sri Lanka. In this latter case, in Sri Lanka and in the Sri Lankan Tamil diaspora, bharata natyam plays a role in the establishment of a shared Tamil identity through, in Sumantra Bose's (1994) terms, a "counter-state" nationalist movement.

In the performance sector, regional concerns articulated themselves differently in the late twentieth century than in the revival. The increasing popularity and renown of other classical Indian dance forms both relied on and queried an association of bharata natyam with nationality. Bharata natyam was the first, but not the only, Indian dance form to be refigured as a classical, urban concert form. It provided a model for dance forms from other regions undergoing their own revival, and reformers of other practices followed the lead set by E. Krishna Iyer and Rukmini Devi (Chatterjea 2004b; Coorlawala 2005). The revival and reconstruction of *odissi* in the 1950s, for example, followed a similar pattern to the recontextualization of bharata natyam (Vatsyayan 1992: 59). Likewise, practitioners brought other regional forms to the concert stage so that states like Andhra Pradesh, Kerala, and Manipur have come to feature their own dance forms.

Therefore, although the bharata natyam revival predated the refiguring of other Indian dance traditions, it contributed to, rather than detracted from, the revival of styles such as *kuchipudi*, *mohini attam*, and *manipuri*. The discursive frame provided by the bharata natyam revival enabled not only the classicizing of existing practices, but also the reconstruction of defunct forms.[13] Outside of

Tamil Nadu, bharata natyam appears alongside rather than replaces forms such as kathak, odissi, and mohini attam. As Uttara Coorlawala argues, the bharata natyam revival put in place a discourse of classicism, defined as accordance with Sanskrit texts, that in turn enabled other classical dance traditions to be "discovered" (1993: 269–70, 1996: 68, 2005: 178). Bharata natyam, thus, is less the national dance of India than the model for the (re-)classicization of India's dance forms.

By the late twentieth century, most regions of India had claimed their own regional, classical form. On the one hand, as Ananya Chatterjea (2004b) argues, this process ushered in a uniform aesthetic that guided efforts at classicization. Chatterjea maintains that the "sculptors of modern Odissi" faced a double bind: to draw out the dance genre's specific traits while also lining it up with the overarching criteria for classicism put in place by the bharata natyam revivalists (2004b: 147–49). Uttara Coorlawala likewise maintains that classicization rested upon a "Sanskritization" of dance practices through pan-Indianist devices used by Rukmini Devi and other dance reformers (2005: 178). On the other hand, the process of discovering, identifying, and reclassicizing these forms highlighted differences in choreographic practice across forms. The competing pulls of national and regional affiliation continued to articulate themselves in the process of uncovering regionally distinct practices that nonetheless shared a set of classical features.

At the same time, bharata natyam retained an ability to operate as a pan-Indian or even pan–South Asian symbol of cultural identity. Dancers, of a range of ethnic and linguistic origins, in all the major cities of India and Sri Lanka study and perform bharata natyam, while the performance of another regional form by a Tamil dancer in Chennai is rare. Similarly, diasporic South Asians, who come from a variety of regional, language, and even religious backgrounds, pursue training in bharata natyam. The celebration of a pan-Indian cultural commonality remains appealing for emigrants because it meets the needs of a transnational, multilingual community for whom regional difference fades in comparison to a threatened assimilation into Western culture. The interweaving of bharata natyam with nationality in this context rests on its operation as a device for "intentional cultural reproduction" (Appadurai 1996). The interest of a global, nonresident Indian community in bharata natyam as a cultural symbol relies upon and reinforces the ability of the dance form to represent this kind of nationhood.

Thus, the production of sociopolitical identity in late-twentieth-century bharata natyam engaged with a burgeoning of separatist regional sentiment in South Asia generally, on the one hand, and with a more harmonious relationship between Tamil and the nation-state in Chennai, on the other. In addition, the imagination of community within late-twentieth-century bharata natyam appeared alongside the visibility of other regional classical dances. National and regional allegiances expressed themselves through bharata natyam's transnational position and its relationship to diasporic identity production. Regional differences diminished when bharata natyam's significance as a diasporic South Asian practice increased. Bharata natyam in the late twentieth century thus veered alternately toward the production of a unified South Asian global identity and the increased specificity of cultural affiliation.

In 1995 the California choreographer Mythili Kumar created a piece entitled *The Life of Gandhi* in anticipation of India's fiftieth anniversary as a sovereign state. In depicting episodes from the life of the legendary activist, the work celebrates a globally recognized version of the Indian nation-state and integrates this history with the movement vocabulary and gestural language of bharata natyam. Here, bharata natyam operates as a vehicle for expressing Gandhi's spiritualization of nationality, a move that echoes the cultural nationalism of Rukmini Devi.

The Life of Gandhi counterposes dramatic episodes and abstract bharata natyam phrases, interweaving the dance form's characteristic mudras with more realistic, full-body theatrical blocking. The work opens with the choreographer appearing in role of Mani Ben, Mohandas Gandhi's grandniece and author of the biography on which the dance is based. She narrates, in English, episodes from Gandhi's life. She begins with Gandhi, as a small child, learning a method for conquering fear that the young Mohandas retained throughout his life. While a thunderstorm rages outside of his home, Gandhi's mother teaches him a sloka for reciting the names of the deities Rama and Sita.

The stage lights come up on a simple domestic interior inhabited by two young female dancers, one clad in a plain sari, the other in boys' clothing of a kurta, or loose, long shirt, and *pyjama* trousers. The sound of thunder and rain crackles over the sound system, and lightning flashes. The boy runs to a corner of the house, quaking in fear. The mother glides to her son and encloses him in her arms. With her left arm encircling her child, she extends her hand to him to get his attention. When he raises his head, she teaches him a recitation. He joins his mother in the chant as musicians sing the verse, "Rama Rama Jaya Sitaram," in praise of Lord Rama and the goddess Sita.

The ensemble files onto the stage. The dancers, hands held in a prayer position, enunciate the verse's rhythm in their walk as they transverse the stage. They launch a unison staccato phrase. Articulate hands cross torsos that tilt and bend over the powerful footwork.

Short vignettes follow one another in this fashion as Mani Ben recounts events from the Mahatma's life that the cast of twelve dancers then embodies, inserting virtuoso rhythmic phrases between narrative sections. The viewer witnesses incidents from Gandhi's childhood and encounters the religious and ethical influences on his upbringing. The tone shifts when the audience learns of Gandhi's first act of nonviolent resistance as he contests segregation rules on a train in South Africa.

As the lights rise, a dancer appears from the wings, wearing Gandhi's signature wire-framed glasses but clad in an elegant Western-style suit and carrying a briefcase. The strength of Gandhi's ethical and political values quickly becomes apparent when he enters a train compartment. Although the wall prominently displays a placard that reads "Whites Only," Gandhi takes a seat. Another dancer, clad in the train conductor's uniform and cap, strides up to Gandhi briskly, points to the sign, and signals the young man to go. Mohandas' polite but clear demur antagonizes the conductor, whose sharp, fast, unfocused gestures contrast with Gandhi's delicate but direct refusal. The conductor's frenzy attracts the attention of other employees and passengers, who join in the fracas. The ensemble converges upon Gandhi, who remains implacable, despite their physical manipulation and abuse. Finally, the mob descends upon him, dragging him from his seat and throwing him from the train.

A subsequent scene portrays not only the Mahatma's fortitude but also his success in transmitting the values of *satyagraha*, or nonviolent resistance. Gandhi, now dressed in his characteristic *khadi*, or homespun cloth, has returned to India. He stands before a multitude, instructing them in the use of oppositional nonviolence against the British imperial government. Gandhi reaches off into the distance, tracing a path with his hand. He bends to the floor with a scooping motion and holds his hand cupped close to his chest. He then traces the return route. A raised index finger close to his torso and a gesture out to the throng indicate the crowd's inclusion in this action. The Dandi Salt March—the protest that inaugurated the nationalist satyagraha movement—has begun.

The group follows Gandhi across the stage. Two dancers in colonial garb and pith helmets, their staffs raised, attempt to guard the sea from which the nationalists will draw salt. The crowd, acting with determination but without aggression, overwhelms them. Their calm torsos over a sharp, articulated walk recall the cast's first ensemble appearance onstage. This time, however, the explosion of rhythmic movements that follows the meditative walk indicates a celebration of victory.

In *The Life of Gandhi*, bharata natyam articulates a nationalist theme. The choreography recounts the Gandhian mission and invokes the activist version of Indian national allegiance that dismantled colonialism. Here, bharata natyam expresses Gandhi's pan-Indianist, spiritualized nationality. By aligning bharata natyam with Gandhi's agenda, Kumar echoes Rukmini Devi's project of highlighting bharata natyam's national significance and augmenting the religious and philosophical meanings of the dance form. Although premiered in 1995, this piece echoes the refiguration of bharata natyam under nationalist auspices in the 1930s.

The Chennai choreographer Lakshmi Viswanathan, by contrast, integrates regional and national histories for bharata natyam in her *Vata Vriksha* or *Banyan Tree*.[14] The piece opens with the choreographer's onstage introduction of "the story of the dance of my people." *Banyan Tree*, its choreography interspersed with Viswanathan's English commentary, traces the history of South Indian dance from ancient folk celebrations to the bharata natyam revival of the 1930s. Although *Banyan Tree* diverges in structure, vocabulary, and thematic content from the conventional items of bharata natyam repertoire, and although it addresses movement forms other than solo classical dance, the narrative treats the vicissitudes of bharata natyam's past as central to its history.[15] The story portrays several devadasi dance contexts, positions the anti-nautch debates as its conflict, and features the refiguration of sadir in the early twentieth century as its crux, achieving its resolution in bharata natyam's emergence on the concert stage.

The piece opens with villagers of the Kaveri River delta dancing to celebrate a successful hunt. When the men return home from their exploits, the women dance in welcome. Creeping in unison, the returning men take broad lunges, displaying the same might and vigor they did during their quest. The women, by contrast, rejoice, dancing with light, rapid footwork and graceful arm movements. They honor the men's success by facing the line of male dancers and arching into deep lunges with arms upraised.

A possession ritual follows. One woman breaks away from the group and thrashes about wildly, whipping her head and upper torso from side to side, her long, unbound hair swinging about her, while the others watch with expressions of awe and fear on their faces. When the entranced woman emerges from this altered state and regains a calm demeanor, she places her hands in the classical mudra for a divine figure: her right hand cupped, palm facing outward, and fingertips lifted, with the left similarly positioned but with the fingertips pointing down. Her serene spiritual power quiets and contains the more disruptive aspects of her transformation.

The ensemble then inducts a young devadasi into temple service. She performs basic exercises before her guru, who sits beside her, keeping time. The devadasi's brief enactment of footwork displays the austerity and discipline of her vocation, after which a sheet is raised to hide the devadasi and a Brahman priest, suggesting her sexual initiation. A more richly attired young woman, the courtesan dancer Madhavi of the epic *Silappadikaram*, enters the stage and bows to her mentor and accompanists. The seriousness with which she crosses the space and the devotion she exhibits toward her teacher suggest that this event marks her entry into professional performance.

The following scene depicts the richness of medieval Thanjavur's cultural life. Craftspeople perform a number of tasks associated with temple arts in an efficient, contented manner. The dancers, for example, suggest the carving of sculpture, tracing lines and curves as their fingers tap along the stone's surface. Outsiders, presumably the Moghuls who conquered the Vijayanagara empire, invade and destroy this utopian society. Dancers hold flexed hands to their mouths in fear. Others extend arms to one side, with their heads turned away from the source of their dismay. The abject citizens collapse to the floor, booming sounds accompanying their falls.

Their debasement constitutes a low point for the temple population. The aesthetic milieu recovers from this devastation, however, for the new rulers, the Nayakas, revive indigenous culture and bring the arts and letters to new heights. Artistic refinement manifests in an ensemble rendition of a classical bharata natyam varnam. Elegantly attired courtiers stand to one side and gaze on appreciatively and attentively.

Again, a period of decline ends this flourish of creativity, with the devadasis experiencing another kind of degradation through sexual subjugation and economic dependence. The dancers sit on the floor in male-female couples. The men encircle the female dancers' waists or shoulders with their arms and touch their faces, both arrogance and desire in their facial expressions. Dance performance does not appear at all in this scene, further indicating the devadasis' artistic decline and their disassociation from their traditional source of both respect and income.

Madras elites take up the devadasis' abandoned artistic project when the temple women fall from favor. This process begins with the debates of the 1920s on the social acceptability of bharata natyam. The dance revivalist E. Krishna Iyer and anti-nautch activist Muttulakshmi Reddy stand off, back to back, with arms folded across their chests as they turn counterclockwise. Rukmini Devi's first encounter with classical dance, through Anna Pavlova's *Dying Swan* solo, follows this unresolved conflict. Pavlova, costumed in diaphanous white, travels across the stage, arms tracing soft and indirect shapes, legs taut and extended, while Rukmini Devi stands to one side and watches, transfixed. When Devi's enchantment with Pavlova encourages her to return to Madras in search of a local dance tradition, however, her endeavors meet with opposition. An elite Madras community reacts with both outrage and intrigue to the news that Devi has begun studying sadir. Sitting on the edge of the stage, they lean toward one another's ears with cupped hands shielding their gossip. Their "secret" reveals itself, however, when their stylized gestures spell out "she dances" while their facial expressions convey their disparagement of Devi's undertaking.

Meanwhile, the performance of an early-twentieth-century dancer continues the devadasi tradition on the concert stage. Although nineteenth-century courtesan dancers epitomized sophistication in their refined stage presence, the twentieth-century dancer, through the *Dhanike Tagujanara* varnam, offers a performance that appears somewhat dated, suggesting that the devadasi tradition has declined further. The narrative returns to Rukmini Devi, whose skillful performance of tasteful classical dances silences her contemporaneous detractors. Her successful concert wins over her gossiping peers. The same public lauds her accomplishment, reversing its opinion and accepting Devi's views on the beauty of dance. They embrace bharata natyam as part of their cultural landscape. The lights come down on an ensemble that celebrates the journey of dance to the present day concert stage.

Lakshmi Viswanathan's *Banyan Tree*, performed for Chennai audiences in 1995 and 1996, offers its viewers the opportunity to identify with the tribulations and triumphs of an imagined community through dance. Language and cultural accomplishment, rather than membership in a political state, define this social group. In order to create an overarching cultural unity, Viswanathan aligns traditions that might otherwise distinguish themselves by intralinguistic differences of location, the social and economic status of their practitioners, and historical period. *Banyan Tree* thereby inspires affinity for and identification with the Tamil people by eliding the practices of discrepant classes and castes with one another.[16] The piece circumvents urban-rural divides, linking village folk practices with the performances of devadasis and, subsequently, of Madras's middle and upper classes in the 1930s and 1940s.

Viswanathan's choreography thus eschews contemporaneous distinctions—and conflicts—between forms identified as folk and classical, elite and subaltern, by collapsing them into a single trajectory. Marginalized peoples do not detract from the consolidation of an urban identity around an elite form. Conversely, lower-caste practices do not define Tamilness to the exclusion of upper-caste ones, as they would in a radical Dravidianist history. Instead, *Banyan Tree* links the marginal strata of society into its dance continuum so that they contribute to the emergence of a highly sophisticated concert art form. *Banyan Tree* positions the bharata natyam revival as the fruit of centuries of all Tamil peoples' choreographic labor.

While Viswanathan foregrounds southern Indian origins and does not look to Sanskrit aesthetic theory or other non-Tamil sources for information on historical dance practices, the narrative provides viewers with the opportunity to identify with the nationalist community that refigured bharata natyam as a concert art form. This conflation of class differences into stages that fuel the bharata natyam revival parallels a strategy, identified by Sally Ness (1997) and Susan Reed (2002), in which nationalists claim subaltern practices as more genuinely precolonial than elite forms because of the latter's contact with colonizers. *Banyan Tree* therefore traces a narrative in which South Indian dance practices merge historically, culminating in E. Krishna Iyer's and Rukmini Devi's recrafting of bharata natyam in the interest of patriotism. *Banyan Tree* characterizes bharata natyam's history as a journey from one imagined community—the region of Tamil Nadu—to another, the nation-state.

The Maharashtrian dancer Sucheta Chapekar offers yet another solution to the question of regional and national affiliation in dance, revisiting a unity-in-diversity (Sethuraman 1985: 46) vision of India through the thematic of language. With the assistance of two mentors, Acharya Parvati Kumar and Kittappa Pillai, Chapekar staged seventeenth- and eighteenth-century dance compositions, written in the Marathi language but performed in the Thanjavur court. She found musical scores written by King Shahaji (1671–1711) at the Saraswati Mahal Library of Thanjavur and, in collaboration with Pillai, choreographed them using the movement vocabulary of present-day bharata natyam.

Sucheta Chapekar's interest in Marathi compositions began under the tutelage of her guru, Parvati Kumar, who researched the compositions of the Maratha King Serfoji II (1793–1832) of Thanjavur. She began her own reconstruction work in the 1970s, offering a lecture-demonstration on this project at the Music Academy in 1971, followed by her first full-length concert of this material in 1974 (Sethuraman 1985: 45). In a 1990 concert at the National Centre for the Performing Arts in Bombay, Chapekar presented these compositions in a solo performance that adhered to the conventional margam. In the abstract dance items, she executed complex staccato phrases, emphasizing the distinctive features of the musical composition, such as, for instance, an alarippu that shifts between five different talas. For dramatic dance items, she translated the Marathi text into the fluid mudras of bharata natyam.

Chapekar has also integrated bharata natyam and Hindustani (North Indian classical) music and through both of these projects she champions a nationalist vision based on regional difference (Sethuraman 1985: 45). Like other bharata natyam practitioners, she presents a version of history that supports her understanding of cultural allegiance. Chapekar, however, refers to a historical period characterized by hybridity rather than seeking in history an origin for a pan-Indian practice. Shahaji, the composer of Chapekar's reconstructed works, was a Maratha ruler from northwest India (now the state of Maharashtria) who ruled southern India from the city of Thanjavur. The Marathas, despite their status as outside occupiers of South India, galvanized indigenous art forms such as sadir and Carnatic music and prompted the development of new performance genres such as the kuravanji (Peterson 1998: 42). Shahaji also supported a multilingual arts milieu, writing and sponsoring dance and music that included Marathi lyrics. The seventeenth- to nineteenth-century Maratha court was itself multilingual and characterized by intercultural experiments including Shahaji's own compositions, modernizing projects in performance and spectatorial protocol, and engagement with colonial music forms (Subramanian 2006). South Indian music, dance, and theater flourished during this period of patronage, stimulated by hybridity and exchange. For Chapekar, the Maratha period provides a model for the harmonious coexistence and cross-fertilization of different cultures, languages, and practices (Sethuraman 1985: 46).

Whereas Rukmini Devi reconstructed an idealized, originary practice that accommodated a shared pan-Indian heritage, Chapekar foregrounds a history where linguistic and cultural legacies converge. Despite her emphasis on Marathi language composition, her strategy parallels that of a Tamil classicist (Ramaswamy 1997) who finds India's great traditions in the historical cross-fertilization of several venerable traditions. Like Balasaraswati, Chapekar locates the origins of this eminent heritage in the city of Thanjavur. However, for Balasaraswati, Thanjavur supported a Tamil legacy, whereas Chapekar sees the city's multilingual and multicultural history as paradigmatic for the contemporary Indian nation. Chapekar therefore argues that Thanjavur exemplified unity in diversity, aligning both the historical city and the dance form it produced with a Nehruvian nationalist vision (in Sethuraman 1985: 46).[17] Moreover, Chapekar's choreography emphasizes not a seamless transition from regional to national associations, as Viswanathan's does, but an intentional return to cross-regional dialogue.

Chapekar's vision of intercultural exchange acquires greater force when seen in the light of the rise of exclusionary regionalism in Maharashtra in the 1990s. As Tamil Nadu has aligned its regionalist discourse increasingly with the nation-state, fragmentary politics gathered strength in Maharashtra. Antagonistic regional and linguistic loyalties emerged in the state in reaction to the increasing cosmopolitanism of the capital city of Bombay (renamed Mumbai in 1996). Hindu fundamentalist and ethnic and linguistic exclusionary organizations such as the Shiv Sena party propagated a xenophobic, communalist definition of cultural and religious allegiance, opposing the immigration of "outsiders" into the relatively prosperous metropole. Chapekar's choreography provides an alternate understanding of regional identity to that proposed by exclusionists because her interpretation of history counters the premise that regional identities inherently counter one another. Her view of the Thanjavur past as one of interchange between equivalent cultural practices contests the claim that regional affiliation opposes linguistic and religious diversity.

Choreographing Tamil Eelam

Whereas Sucheta Chapekar describes bharata natyam as a product of cross-cultural exchange, the Toronto choreographer Vasu presents it as a tool for ending subjugation. Vasu originally hails from the Jaffna region of Sri Lanka. He teaches bharata natyam under the auspices of the Tamil Eelam Society, a Toronto-based organization that exists primarily to provide social services for Tamil refugees but that also, as its name implies, embraces a "counter-state nationalist" (Bose 1994) view of the Sri Lankan political situation.[18] Vasu, in his choreography, expresses views similar to those of the organization that supports his work. In 1999, he produced a dance drama entitled *Vilangukal Sidaiyum Kalam* (*When the Chains Are Broken*) that charts, through bharata natyam, the trials of the Tamil people. His students performed this piece for the Tamil Eelam Society's July 1999 Karumpulikal Nal (Black Tigers Day), which commemorates the suicide commandos of the Liberation Tigers of Tamil Eelam (LTTE).

Vilangukal Sidaiyum Kalam, like *Banyan Tree*, opens with an ensemble that depicts Tamil folk dance traditions. Children and young teens, clad as villagers, use bharata natyam's hand gestures but inflect the classical form's solid footwork with a light buoyancy to suggest rural dances. With articulate hands and arms, they portray the peasants' agricultural chores. The bucolic tone shifts dramatically when another group races out from the wings and descends upon the Tamil villagers. Their fierce slashing motions and frightening expressions scatter the country folk, who huddle in fear until the marauding hordes dissipate.[19]

The next scene takes place several centuries later. The cast appears in elaborate eighteenth-century European costumes, with girls in wide skirts and boys in rich velvet coats. Genteelly bowing to one another, they form pairs and waltz across the stage. Their positioning in male-female couples and their foreign costumes signal that they have brought an alien culture with them. The villagers, however, absent themselves during this scene, suggesting that the British ruled from a distance.

The British appear civilized, if arrogant, but the next invaders, the Sinhalese, are terrifying. The following scene opens with the Tamil people reaccessing their cultural glories. The townspeople, now more refined than agricultural, exhibit their cultural pride by flanking an ornately bejeweled woman. Her crown, rich attire, and raised palm indicate that she is Tamil Tay, or Mother Tamil, a goddesslike figured described in Tamil language politics as the embodiment of Tamil culture (Ramaswamy 1997). Regal in her demeanor, she stands surrounded by her awed and devoted subjects.

Sinhalese soldiers, complete with the fatigues and weaponry of a modern military force, swoop onto the stage, scattering the townsfolk. They swagger about the stage, confident that they have broken the will of the populace. The soldiers approach Tamil Tay, who no longer has the protection of her people, and drag her to a prison cell on the opposite side of the stage.[20] Although the Tamil people's despair manifests itself in their wringing hands and drooped postures, all is not lost. Another group, clad in the black fatigues and berets of the Tamil Tigers' suicide commando brigade, bursts from the wings. Their thundering footwork shatters the complacency of the Sinhalese soldiers, whom they easily overwhelm. They release Tamil Tay from her prison, and the ensemble performs a joyous dance.

Vasu's work is part of a larger phenomenon. In the 1990s, Sri Lankan Tamil choreographers, both in Jaffna and internationally, created pieces that expressed separatist nationalism and that celebrated the efforts of the LTTE to create an independent Tamil nation. Not surprisingly, this period, in which dancers produced choreography that foregrounded nationalist sentiment, also witnessed the escalation of the war between the Sri Lankan military and the LTTE. This staging of counter-state dances was not a fringe venture: when the LTTE controlled the Jaffna peninsula in the mid-1990s, they sponsored this type of choreography in festivals and competitions (Mahendra personal correspondence 2004). In Canada, the Tamil nationalist television program *Oliveechu*, based on a contraband radio program of the same name in Sri Lanka, included such pieces alongside its news reports on the war. This contribution to the Black Tiger commemoration supports the crafting of Tamil counter-state nationalism through choreography.

Vilangukal Sidaiyum Kalam draws together the history and symbolism of Tamil Nadu and the putative Tamil Eelam, positioning bharata natyam alongside historical invasions and the glories that Tamil Tay represents as a cultural link between these two regions. The work follows a structure similar to Viswanathan's piece in that it depicts successive waves of invasions and posits that Tamil identity emerged out of its recuperation from these conquests. Unlike Viswanathan, however, Vasu does not integrate bharata natyam with the existing nation-state. He does not follow Kumar's approach of affiliating bharata natyam with pan-national spiritual traditions, of either India or Sri Lanka. And in contrast to Chapekar, he does not join together different regional traditions. Instead, in Vasu's choreography, bharata natyam expresses a Tamil cultural affiliation to the exclusion of other associations. The dance form provides a means not of resolving regional and language differences through national unity, but of demonstrating the need for a separate nation-state based on linguistic and ethnic commonality.

Although Vasu's piece treats bharata natyam solely as an emblem of Tamil cultural identity, it nonetheless follows the lead of early-twentieth-century practitioners such as Iyer and Devi by using the dance form to represent national identity. In its challenge to the authority of the Sri Lankan government, the piece does not dispute the idea of the nation-state in general, nor does it question bharata natyam's ability to represent nationhood. Instead, through bharata natyam, Vasu stakes out a claim for the legitimacy of a new nation: Tamil Eelam. Although Vasu projects a separatist allegiance instead of the metropolitan nationalism of practitioners such as Rukmini Devi, he uses bharata natyam as a means of mobilizing nationalist sentiment.

Vasu's piece addresses not only the Sri Lankan situation of the 1990s, but also the position of Tamil Canadians. For this community, counter-state nationalism not only challenges the legitimacy of the Sri Lankan government but also contributes to ethnic identity in diaspora. In international contexts, separatist movements such as the Tamil Eelam struggle draw their legitimacy from an ideology of nationhood in exile. As Verne Dusenberry (1995) argues, ethnic identity in multicultural societies relies upon the idea of the nation, especially in countries such as Canada that reject an assimilation ideal and celebrate cultural difference. This expression of nationalism therefore contributes to the production of immigrant identity as much as to a new nation-state.

Although *Vilangukal Sidaiyum Kalam* uses a mixed-gender cast, most Tamil separatist choreographies represent their nationalist sentiment through performances by girls and young women. Because the pool of available dancers is predominantly female and because the LTTE has not only accepted but also actively recruited women soldiers, female dancers portray the actions of the LTTE, taking the roles of male and female combatants on both sides of the conflict. The role of young women in these dance dramas conjoins with the dual function that bharata natyam performs for emigrant Sri Lankan Tamil communities: a means of expressing nationalist sentiment and a device for preserving Tamil culture. This dual function relies upon a conflation, in Sri Lanka, of bharata natyam with both femininity and with Tamil national identity. Tamil separatist choreographies, although they diverge from their Indian counterpoints in their understanding of national and regional identity, depend on the same intersection of femininity, nationalism, and cultural reproduction that, as I shall argue in the next chapter, practitioners of the revival introduced.

Vasu's composition brings into relief concerns of gender and transnationalism as well as of regionalism and nationality. Bharata natyam, as a symbol of imagined communities, enables its practitioners either to resolve tensions between the nation and region or to posit new, more specific definitions of political identity. Dancers created such affiliations through discourses of gender and feminine respectability as well as through cultural and linguistic associations. Likewise, practitioners contended with bharata natyam's transition to new environments and contexts of performance. Thus, bharata natyam provides a vehicle for imagining community not only through language, history, and allegiance to a homeland but also, as I shall indicate in the next chapters, through gender and through the consolidation of local identities.

3: Women's Questions

The Home and the World: Reinventing the Feminine in Indian Colonial Politics

Bharata natyam appears at first glance to be an overtly feminine practice. Although men perform both solo and in ensemble dances, they remain in the minority and are celebrated for their exceptional status. More significantly, the choreography reads as feminine, with its lyrical grace, its elaborate costuming and make-up, and, in some renditions, its coy and flirtatious glances. This last girlish or coquettish stage presence nonetheless appears contained, even innocent. The gendering of bharata natyam thus intertwines visual pleasure with an enduring sense of propriety.[1]

This appealing yet respectable femininity did not grow up organically out of the dance practice or out of the marginal sexual and domestic lives of devadasi practitioners. An association of women and sensuality with bharata natyam developed, in the first instance, alongside the complex gender investments of the bhakti movement and its literary products. Revival-era dancers then addressed the gender concerns of performance in negotiation with their perception of the devadasi tradition. The more specific intersection of reputability with pleasing spectacle developed through a series of debates around the role of dance in the life of the women of the Indian nation. Likewise, it emerged from conflicting political points of view about the status of Indian women. Just as performers and promoters inserted dance into nationalist discourse, as an emblem of cultural pride, they also engaged, through performance, with debates over femininity, respectability, and gender subjugation in Indian cultural practices. As in the case of definitions of tradition, discourses of creativity, and questions of cultural allegiance, these competing ideas around the role of dance, women, class, and nationhood descended, in the first instance, from the complexities of indigenous gender paradigms, and subsequently from the colonial encounter and its nationalist responses.

British colonialists in India defended their imperial venture on the grounds that the "civilizing mission" uplifted "debased natives" and saved them from their own restrictive traditions. Through this ideology, imperialists insisted that the abject status of Indian women and other "vulnerable" members of society persisted not because of the actions of individuals but through the sanction of tradition (Chatterjee 1993: 118). Colonialists further maintained that these social inequities illustrated the unfitness of Indians to rule themselves and the resultant need for imperial intervention (Spivak 1988: 297; Rajan 1993: 42). Colonizers thereby justified imperial rule through reference to the subjugation of Indian women. In doing so, as Lata Mani argues, they rendered women neither agents nor even objects of social action, but rather symbols of India, of a society in need of reform (1990: 98, 117).

Such censure emphasized the inequities of Indian society on its most basic levels. As a result, early- to mid-nineteenth-century activism in India focused as much on societal issues as governmental ones. Public agitations divided between the imperative to reform or revive cultural traditions and social practices. Reformists sought to alter Indian society so that it more closely accommodated modern European ideals of equality. Revivalists, by contrast, underscored the merits of orthodox Indian Hindu culture. They saw the status of women as validating India's ancient cultural practices and as therefore legitimizing the would-be nation-state. Revivalists could not completely circumvent colonial condemnation, so they strove to access the values of an ancient, presumably more egalitarian Indian past (Chakravarti 1990). Individual nationalists affiliated themselves with one camp or the other, calling for reform so that India could merit freedom or resisting societal transformation as a colonial incursion into Indian culture. Women's position in society, for several oppositional sets—nationalists and colonialists, reformists and revivalists—served as a benchmark of civilization.

By the late nineteenth century, as Partha Chatterjee argues, nationalists of both groups redirected the woman question to the creation of the iconic *bhadramahila*, or "respectable lady" (1993: 116–32), India's "new woman," who combined the merits of tradition with a forward-looking embrace of progressive values. Nationalists concerned with feminine reputability resorted to revivalist discourse when they maintained that "traditional" society offered women both a valued standing and protection. They conflated the indigenous *sumangali*, or auspicious woman—virtuous, self-sacrificing, yet replete with spiritual power—and the ideal Victorian woman, who enjoyed a complementary difference from her companionate spouse (Roy 1998: 129). Although this iconic figure developed out of the values of orthodox Indian domestic norms and thus in accord with revivalist ideals, the model bhadramahila also accommodated reformist critique, for she would be educated and would exercise volition. The new respectable lady thus differed from uneducated lower-class women, who inhabited the public sphere by necessity, and from the previous generation of elite women, who were constrained by tradition rather than mobilized in its interest (Chatterjee 1993: 127, 129). In exchange for traditional respect combined with new freedom, the bhadramahila would preserve India's cultural heritage in the domestic realm and embody its values. Furthermore, respectable women were to salvage tradition in order to compensate for the compromise with colonial culture that the outside world demanded of men (126).

As Chatterjee argues, nationalist discourses divided lived experience into the two categories of "home" and "the world," or *ghar* and *bahir*. These terms, like the word bhadramahila, are Bengali, indicating the extent to which the reform and revival movements and their nationalist "resolution" emerged out of the early- to mid-nineteenth-century Bengali renaissance. These two spheres supported both gender and national differences, lining up with a set of oppositions: "the home" accorded with women, tradition, and "the East," while "the world" aligned with men, modernity, and "the West" and its colonial realms. Women upheld the values of the home, while men participated in the culturally hybrid domain of the outside world. The home remained the domain of the spiritual, traditional "East," while the world belonged to the material, dynamic "West." Nationalists, unlike colonialists, depicted spirituality and tradition as sources of strength rather than weakness. When these two sets of binaries came together, the spirituality of the East would triumph within the "uncolonized," feminine realm of the home and its practices (119–21), even while the West retained its dominance in the exterior, material space of the world.[2] Although these concepts emerged from nineteenth-century Bengali activism, they facilitated the ideological tactics of nationalists and regionalists in Tamil Nadu.

Nationalists located a number of arenas in which the distinction between home and world could articulate itself. For instance, as Chatterjee indicates, in order to distinguish the bhadramahila from lower-class, Westernized, and orthodox women, nationalists reconstructed dress as a symbol of an authentic yet new nationality. A fundamental distinction in Indian society of the nineteenth and early twentieth centuries permitted men to adopt European clothes (trousers, shirts, and shoes) while requiring women to dress in a "traditional" manner. However, the now standard urban middle-class woman's outfit—a sari worn with petticoat, blouse, and shoes—developed out of experiments in the nineteenth century with colonial and indigenous attire. Chatterjee therefore suggests that it is itself hybrid (1993: 130). This ensemble inscribed the virtues of the "home"—femininity and essential Indianness—while also representing a break from the past. This characteristic dress became the norm of Indian feminine attire that contrasted with the Western apparel worn by middle-class men until the Gandhian agitations of the twentieth century. Post-independence, this distinction reemerged, with men adopting European clothing and urban middle-class women retaining the sari combination. Thus, dress consolidated a female identity that incorporated both tradition and reform, distinguishing middle-class "respectable" women both from their predecessors and from their Westernized counterparts.

This split found form in physical and aesthetic practices as well. The identification of cricket as a nationalist activity, for example, operated through its gendering. Cricket, played on a professional level as a marker of India's cultural and political identity and enjoyed on an avocational level by boys and young men of all communities, religions, and locations, is masculine, overtly hybrid, and cross-class (Appadurai 1996). By contrast, "feminine" practices lined up with conventional local ones, emerging, for instance, in classical music, reformed folk traditions, and classical dance. In constructing this interior realm of tradition, nationalists reformed women's activities as much as they claimed them as cultural symbols. They revamped artistic forms that, although associated with feminine domains, did not express appropriate values of modesty and legitimate religiosity. Sumanta Bannerjee analyzes nineteenth-century Bengali popular culture as an example of this phenomenon, arguing that middle-class nationalists restricted and reformed the bawdy, stark songs of marketplace women and Vaishnava performers, having found the cross-class interactions between performers and viewers and the erotic and jocular songs of lower-class women poets, singers, and dancers threatening to new definitions of classical culture (1990: 131–32). They rejected these forms of women's popular culture, demonstrating that some feminine vocations were more accepted than others. For metropolitan nationalists, the feminine realm of the "home" and its tradition required modification and reform as well as preservation.

Nationalists did not limit their modifications to performance and other symbolic practices. Rather, they accepted legislation and social change that altered some aspects of Hindu family and public life, such as those concerning child marriage, widow immolation, and female education. In these instances, nationalists acquiesced to changes that brought Indian practices in line with the norms of the West. However, as Chatterjee argues, nationalists admitted reforms that accorded with their understanding of a public-private divide. They agreed to changes that did not threaten the sovereignty of the bourgeois domestic sphere and that retained or furthered the division of social behavior into indigenous, spiritual, and feminine versus hybrid, material, and masculine practices and traits (Chatterjee 1993: 126).

As a result of these and other social and legislative changes, colonialism is sometimes represented as benefiting women. However, colonial and nationalist reformers sought primarily to bring Indian cultural practices into line with those of Europe, rather than to emancipate women. These maneuvers improved the position of women in some contexts but worsened it in others, abolishing traditional Indian practices that offered women freedom as well as those that oppressed them. Colonial reform movements helped to eradicate such family arrangements as those of devadasis and of castes such as the Nairs of Kerala, in which women controlled their own economic resources, had relative sexual freedom, or retained influence in their homes after marriage as they continued to live with their natal families. Reformers also critiqued the eroticism of bhakti, a tradition that had provided women with public roles as singers, poets, and dancers and thus allowed some women a level of autonomy. More perniciously, colonialists also reified institutions through which women were subjugated. For instance, as Lata Mani (1990) argues, the British colonial interest in establishing the legality of sati served to validate the practice by identifying volition as the key to the legitimacy of widow immolation.

By the late nineteenth century, the division of middle-class life into the spheres of home and the world had presented itself in increasingly figurative terms (Roy 1998: 129). Nationalists transferred the qualities of home—spirituality, traditionalism, cultural authenticity, and sexual propriety—onto elite women themselves. The middle-class lady's responsibility for tradition extended to her incorporating into her own demeanor the home's spiritual and moral values. Paradoxically, this assured that women could move into the public sphere as long as their behavior demonstrated an allegiance to these virtues. Women of the urban middle class pursued formal education, undertook political activism, and eventually took up paid employment because the symbolic markers they adopted, in dress, conduct, and diet, assured that they retained their feminine essence and continued their roles within the patriarchal family (Chatterjee 1993: 130; Roy 1998: 129). This shift from literal to metaphorical domesticity offered elite women liberties that distinguished them from the previous generation of women. At the same time, it ensured that they remained subject to a new framework of patriarchal norms.

Reform and Revival: Bharata Natyam's Contentions over Respectable Womanhood

Partha Chatterjee (1993) argues that the refiguring of elite womanhood resolved the "woman question" and that the emergence of the bhadramahila model of respectable femininity accounts for the seemingly sudden disappearance of gender concerns from nationalist agendas in the late nineteenth century. In other words, the nationalist gendering of separate spheres, according to Chatterjee, allowed the woman question to fade from public life by the late nineteenth century. Although Chatterjee's arguments draw on examples from Bengal, their insights apply to the early-twentieth-century refiguration of bharata natyam, which parallels this process of contention, standardization, reform, and apparent completion. The dance revival relied upon the refiguration and domestication of women's practices. Upper-caste dancers and promoters aligned bharata natyam with the values of reformed spirituality and classicism. Subsequently, middle-class women moved into the public realm of dance performance without compromise to their propriety. So successful was this refiguration that by the post-revival period, dance practice had not only ceased to threaten feminine propriety, it had come to confirm it.[3] Bharata natyam thereby shifted from a "public woman's" form into a public representation of symbolic domesticity through its performance of tradition and spirituality.[4] As they did for activism and employment, these values, once embedded in choreography, enabled middle-class "family women" to enter the arena of dance study and performance without compromising their respectability. Therefore, as Amrit Srinivasan (1983, 1985) argues, the recontextualization of bharata natyam relied upon a conflation of reformist and revivalist agendas and through them articulated a nationalist identity. The bharata natyam revival, like the establishment of the model bhadramahila, consolidated divergent discourses: a marginal women's dance form emerged as a vehicle for the consolidation of iconic femininity.

So important was the incorporation of these gender discourses that the dance form's refiguration as a reputable woman's practice served to undergird its nationalist potential. Bharata natyam's "national" status emerged less from a nationwide prevalence or predominance and more from an ability to express ostensibly ubiquitous Indian middle-class values. Although these values included recourse to Sanskrit aesthetic theory and to pan-Indian epics, as indicated in chapter 2, they also relied on a reformed version of (elite Hindu) female identity. Bharata natyam's popularity in the post-revival period among middle-class Indians inside and outside of Tamil Nadu rested on revival-era practitioners' success in intertwining the dance form with nationalist strategies of gender construction. The representation of bharata natyam as symbolic of the "domestic" values of tradition, classicism, religiosity, and spirituality allowed the dance practice to function as a symbol of pan-Indian, and, in some cases, pan–South Asian middle-class feminine propriety.[5]

This process was neither unqualified nor uncontested, however. The status of the amateur adolescent dancer, for instance, as a proper and traditional young lady exemplified the dance form's function as a marker, albeit a glamorized one, of heritage, religion, and classicized culture. By contrast, the professional performance of dance, especially for mature women, compromised these resonances of symbolic domesticity. For many women, even in the late twentieth century, public performance remained an unacceptable option because of bharata natyam's enduring association with nondomestic sexuality and because it carried with it demands from outside the home. This was particularly true for married women who incurred their families' disapproval if they continued their concert appearances. Some professional dancers remained unmarried in order to be able to continue their performance career without incurring the disapproval of a marital family, while others upon marriage shifted their emphasis toward teaching. Other women performed publicly but distanced themselves from the term professional dancer.

Because the domestication of bharata natyam remained partial, nationalist gender discourses, with their contrasting reformist and revivalist positions, endured from the late nineteenth century into the twentieth. As such, the refiguration of bharata natyam contrasts with the nationalist discourse discussed by

Chatterjee. The respectability of bharata natyam remained unstable well into the twentieth century with dancers, promoters, and critics defending the form through reference to its history and its cultural significance. In doing so, they voiced reformist and revivalist positions as they related to dance. Moreover, the revival of bharata natyam allowed a new generation of dancers to carve out authoritative subject positions through the representation of the dance form and its tradition. In order to defend their practice of a marginal form, they reclaimed or circumvented the devadasi legacy, treating it at once as their origin and their "other."

Thus, as Gayatri Spivak argues in reference to the Anglo-American literary critical attempt to recover female subjectivities, the representation of "others" facilitated the establishment of subject positions (1999: 113–14, 116–17). Discourses of reform and revival and their concomitant representation of "others" endured in twentieth-century bharata natyam because they remained productive for the consolidation of subject positions. The title of this chapter, then, plays on the expected meanings of "the woman question:" on the one hand, the woman question, as raised within nationalism, positioned women as objects of reform and as images of India, subsequently figuring them as emblems and protectors of tradition. On the other hand, the bharata natyam revival refigured and realigned nationalist gender discourses so that, through them, the new generation of practitioners established their own authoritative stance on the dance form, raising questions about the tradition and their role in it.

The incomplete nature of this resolution descends from the anti-nautch controversy, which complicated the domestication of femininity in choreography. In the late nineteenth century—the same time that Chatterjee finds a resolution of the women's question in nationalist discourse in Bengal—the anti-nautch movement launched its agitations for gender reform in southern India. The contrasts between the anti-nautch campaign and the early-nineteenth-century reforms that Chatterjee discusses are manifold. The anti-nautch movement began in southern India in 1892, about fifty years after the other reform agitations. The debate hinged on the status of non-elite women, while the social reform agendas of the early nineteenth century focused on issues such as widow immolation, widow remarriage, child marriage, kulin Brahman polygamy, and female education that affected upper-caste women (Bannerjee 1990: 145–46). Unlike these other agitations, the mobilization against devadasi dedication threatened nothing essential to mainstream Hindu society, especially since the devadasi system had already declined.[6] Although rooted in similar concerns to, for instance, the crusade against child marriage, the anti-nautch movement offered a different solution from that given for the latter campaign: activists addressed the exploitation of girls and women through temple dedication by striving to eradicate the devadasi system rather than to modify it.

In contrast to the early nineteenth century reform movements, such as the legislation against sati and the age of consent controversy, the anti-nautch movement consolidated itself around the efforts of British missionaries and urban Indians, not of British government officials. Indeed, anti-nautch reformers railed against the colonial government for its reluctance to pass anti-dedication legislation. The British government resisted banning the dedication of women to temple service because of its policy of noninterference in matters of native religious life following the 1857 uprising. The anti-nautch movement both began with a different set of assumptions and sparked a different reaction than efforts to reform upper-caste Indian family life.

Nonetheless, these agitations relied upon similar gender values to those of the earlier reform movements. The concerns of the anti-nautch movement accorded with those of other campaigns in that they fixed a specific set of gender norms as they maintained and extended the polarization of male and female roles. Like the earlier colonial reform movements, anti-nautch activists treated devadasis, the target of reform, as symbols of cultural degradation and evaluated their status through colonial ideas of propriety and equality (Srinivasan 1983, 1985; Coorlawala 1996). Reformers urged, for temple dancers, not social and economic autonomy, but a more respectable form of dependence through marriage. As a result, this movement eradicated family structures that did not accord with European and high caste models of domesticity and, like other reform agitations, enhanced gender distinctions.

In this campaign, Victorian feminism blended with a nineteenth-century European sentimentality that tied women's ideal roles to their inherent virtue. Devadasis, according to this argument, were necessarily oppressed as they were systemically denied the domesticity most suited to their feminine "nature." Here, the concern lay with eradicating the cultural sanction on courtesanship, not abolishing extradomestic sexuality generally. Reformers therefore concerned themselves as much with standardizing feminine behavior as with abolishing the subjugation of women, referencing Victorian norms of behavior (Srinivasan 1983: 86) and ostensibly universal standards of morality (Jordan 1989: 4, 167, 205) in order to form their critique. They likewise validated their own political claims, confirming their modernity by applying post-Enlightenment ideas to Indian social life and retaining a dominant discourse on gender and female sexuality.[7]

Despite this shared gender ideology, however, the divergent groups within the anti-nautch campaign held different assumptions and goals. As in the case of regionalist movements, these camps used the anti-nautch movement to different ends in terms of reestablishing gender norms. Muttulakshmi Reddy's arguments conflated feminism and Victorian gender values. Reddy spearheaded the move for anti-dedication legislation, through the Madras Devadasis Prevention of Dedication Bill of 1930, expressing concerns that devadasis could not choose their occupations, remained dependent on men, and were sexually exploited. Nonetheless, she maintained that the proper role of women lay in lifelong monogamous, companionate marriages rather than in complete independence. As a physician, she also contributed to a medicalization of the devadasi controversy, justifying her agitations for reform through scientific concerns about the "health of the race" (in Srinivasan 1983: 82). Reddy argued for women's right to individual volition but simultaneously restricted women's choices to options within the realm of upper-class Victorian and Brahmanical sexual mores.

British missionaries also expressed concerns over women's rights but conjoined them with an intolerance of practices outside of European Protestantism. For them, the devadasis system was abhorrent not only because of its putative immorality, but also because of the respected status offered to dancers by mainstream Indian society. They used this "debased" position of Indian women as a platform for arguing against the British government's noninterference policy.

Indian upper-caste nationalists and urban professionals both generalized their own community's social mores regarding gender and sexuality and were influenced by Christian morality (Srinivasan 1985) when they spoke out against the devadasi system. For these activists, the justification of colonialism through the status of women meant that the extradomestic sexuality of the devadasis contradicted nationalist claims to sovereignty. Conversely, reform and standardization of women's behavior would validate Indian society and would therefore form part of the case they made for national independence.

The non-Brahman regionalist activists, who came to dominate anti-nautch agitations by the 1920s also relied upon European and, ironically, Brahmanical notions of propriety. However, they engaged in these debates in order to offset the disparagement of their communities by disassociating themselves from the devadasi tradition. As indicated in chapter 2, the men of these groups improved their own status, both socially and economically, by bringing their community's family structures in line with colonial and high-caste norms of propriety and by shifting power and economic control within the family from women to men (Srinivasan 1985: 1873, 1874).

As in the case of other reform movements, the anti-nautch movement encountered resistance from revivalists, who defended the devadasi system, usually in terms that simultaneously justified indigenous patriarchy. Few argued that courtesanship deserved consideration as a legitimate set of sexual and domestic practices. Rather, revivalists countered the reformist claim that nondomestic sexuality inhered in devadasi dedication and in dance practice.

Anti-nautch campaigners concerned themselves not only with the status, lifestyle, and social organization of devadasi communities, but also with their dance, especially its dramatic content. They maintained that the devadasi repertoire, especially its erotic idioms, accorded with and contributed to the extradomestic status of its practitioners. They argued that the devadasis' roles as courtesans abased them by relegating them to a life of vice and that their dance practice accorded with their lascivious lifestyle. The controversy conflated the simultaneously pitiable and threatening status of its courtesan practitioners with the dance practice itself and its ostensibly prurient content.

The dramatic content of the dance, and specifically its portrayal of religious sentiment through erotic idioms, developed out of the bhakti movement. Bhakti locates spiritual attainment in a personal allegiance to and affection for a particular god. Its poems emphasize interior experience, exploring a single dramatic moment in all its complexity rather than tracking narrative action. The bulk of bhakti poetry, as used in dance, expresses religious longing through idioms of amatory desire. Moments of contact with the divine compare with the rapture of sexual union. These moments consume the senses and the emotions but dissipate and are quickly relegated to the past. The narrator, who is also usually the main female character, longs for the return of the god-lover and remembers their moments of erotic contact. She speaks of her emotional anxiety, recalling their interaction and describing the effect that elements in the natural environment have on her inflamed senses as she waits for her lover's return. The heroine, although piqued by her lover's inconsistencies, usually relents once he returns his attention to her.[8] Bhakti poetry privileges a female point of view but expresses religious devotion through the longing and frustration of a female character whose class status limits her to a state of helpless inaction. Bhakti role-playing, then, while privileging the perspective of a female character, fixes gender subordination by treating heterosexual intimacy as a metaphor for the innately unequal relationship of a devotee to god.

However, devotionalism also challenged social conventions. The bhakti movement departed from the renunciatory traditions that had preceded it and located the path to enlightenment not in the practice of austerities but in a personal, ecstatic relationship with a particular god. It allowed an egalitarian interpretation of religion by not just accepting but often taking as exemplary the devotion of women, the lower castes, and tribal non-Hindus. By situating spiritual enlightenment in an individual's experience of love for a specific god, devotionalism circumvented the orthodoxy of temple rituals and its accompanying class, caste, and gender hierarchies. Through the bhakti movement, women gained autonomy as they assumed occupations as poets, singers, and dancers of devotional pieces. Especially in the case of the female bhakti poets, devotionalism offered the possibility for women to leave domestic life and escape dependence on men. Bhakti presented bharata natyam with a complex gender legacy in which the poetry treated female characters as paradigmatic and foregrounded their emotions and desires and the tenets of the movement allowed women public roles as devotees, authors, and performers. At the same time, however, these poems expressed religious devotion through stereotypical images of an infatuated and pining heroine.

The anti-nautch movement masked the complex sociopolitical implications of bhakti by emphasizing primarily its explicit treatment of eroticism. The questions raised by the anti-nautch movement regarding the acceptability of sensuality as a metaphor for religious devotion emerged from another colonial conflict: that between the multiplicity of Hindu religious traditions and British Protestantism. Missionaries opposed polytheism generally as well as the representation and worship of gods in iconographic form, condemning the latter as idolatry. British reformers expressed shock at the praise of gods in songs and dances that addressed them playfully and angrily as well as lovingly and that drew out their human, and specifically amorous, qualities. Anti-nautch agitations thus queried the validity of dance that expressed religious experience through sexual metaphors as much as they highlighted the apparently negative social and moral attributes of devadasi social organization and family structures. In doing so, they conflated choreographic content with the sexuality of its practitioners. The relatively marginal standing of devadasis, combined with the representation of eroticism in bhakti songs, meant that the domestication of bharata natyam was partial and less stable than the reform of other feminine practices (Meduri 1996: 334, 398).

Because the anti-nautch movement did not secure legislation banning the dedication of women to temple service until 1947, debates about devadasis coincided with the bharata natyam revival (Srinivasan 1985). Issues raised by anti-nautch activists therefore entered discussions about the recontextualization of bharata natyam as an urban, middle-class practice. When women of "good families" turned to bharata natyam, they embraced and reformed a feminine practice that, through its performance of tradition and spirituality, could represent symbolic domesticity and, hence, national culture. Elite women recrafted bharata natyam into an emblem of the nation, and subsequently the dance form's new status as a national treasure confirmed the propriety and traditionalism of middle-class girls and women. That upper-caste, middle-class dancers performed much of the same choreography as devadasis, including some of its erotic idioms, however, vexed the anti-nautch movement's standardization of gendered practices and behaviors (Srinivasan 1983: 96). These stage appearances threatened even the most persuasive figurations of elite womanhood as representative of a domesticated, national culture.

The anti-nautch movement, with its contestations over gender, class, traditional practices, and sexuality, set the stage for bharata natyam's emergence as an emblem of a reformed classical culture. It both contributed to and complicated the ability of the middle-class, upper-caste bharata natyam dancer to represent feminine respectability, tradition, and symbolic domesticity. The devadasi dancer, who supposedly embodied the negative traits of a public woman, emerged through these contentions both as a foil to the respectable woman and as the self she might become if she were not vigilant.[9] On the one hand, the devadasi legacy established bharata natyam's ability to represent figurative domesticity by acting as its opposite: an entity in need of reform. On the other hand, the status of devadasi performers also threatened the respectable woman's universality (Meduri 1996: 334, 398). In contrast to the early-nineteenth-century reform movements, the anti-nautch campaign left the "women's question" that was embedded in the devadasi controversy incompletely resolved. Questions of reform and revival, as they pertained to dance, continued to be raised into the twentieth century.

The group of practitioners that entered the dance field in the 1930s responded to anti-nautch criticism by mobilizing and querying reform and revival discourses, thereby putting to use already existing claims around gender. In doing so, they established their influence on the dance form, not only through recourse to history, but also specifically through their positions on gendered reform, cultural revivalism, and symbolic domesticity. The new urban middle-class and upper-caste practitioners established their own means of self-representation through reformist and revivalist takes on choreographic practice, crafting a subject position that allowed them to interlocute for the form and its tradition. These strategies of representation facilitated their interlocution for others, especially the devadasi practitioners, who had been pushed to the margins of the dance milieu.

Revival-era dancers structured their own position in the bharata natyam field by deciding how much of the devadasi legacy to maintain and how to legitimize elements of past practice, as well as by identifying areas of traditional praxis that required reform. They occluded particular features of devadasi performance while celebrating others. This extraction of some elements at the expense of others rendered devadasi practice the terrain upon which elite practitioners crafted their representation. The refiguration of sadir as bharata natyam drew together nationalist gender norms, reformist discourses, class issues, and subject constitution, which, in turn, required choreographic reiteration because the "erasure" (Roach 1989) of the disreputable "other" was only partial.

Paradoxically, it was the choreographic practice of E. Krishna Iyer, a male dancer, that initiated this convergence of femininity, respectability, and subjectivity. Iyer directly opposed Muttulakshmi Reddy's campaign to eradicate devadasi dedication and performance. Along with the revivalists, Iyer argued that devadasis deserved credit for perpetuating indigenous classical forms. Like other Madras-based nationalists, he urged the promotion of traditional forms in the interest of indigenous cultural pride, supporting concerts by devadasi practitioners.

Yet Iyer played a different role in the bharata natyam renaissance from his colleagues in patronage and promotion in that he studied and performed sadir himself, presenting items of conventional repertoire clad in devadasi attire and occasionally passing himself off as a hereditary dancer. This cross-gender and cross-class mimicry appears, initially, to contradict the perceived femininity of bharata natyam.[10] However, Iyer's project helped to establish bharata natyam as a respectable, feminine activity by refiguring discourses of gendered reform and revival. He therefore established a pathway through which the dance form could

Figure 14: E. Krishna Iyer. Courtesy: Sruti / Samudri Archives, Chennai.

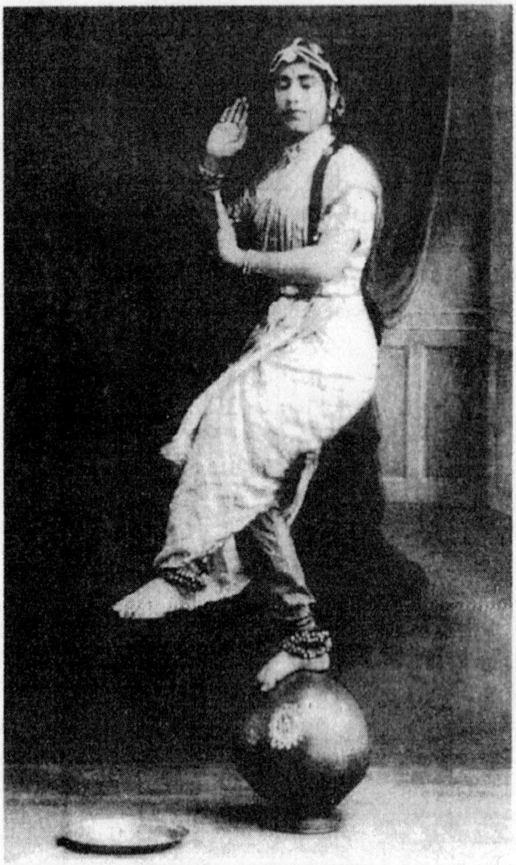

intersect with a revised version of proper womanhood, remade through metropolitan nationalism.

Iyer's discursive position on both nationalism and dance was largely revivalist in that he argued for the preservation of the practices of the past. In his performances, however, he grappled with the competing demands of restoration and reform. On the one hand, he retained much of the devadasi repertoire and performance style. On the other hand, he modified elements associated with the devadasi legacy, such as humorous interludes and spectacular display (Arudra 1986–87d: 33). His revivalist agenda positioned indigenous tradition within women's practices, while his reforms privileged spirituality over humor and devotion over eroticism. By blending nationalism and the purification of tradition in his cross-gender impersonations, he yoked femininity to a refigured classical culture. These tactics, although rooted in a celebration of the devadasi tradition, established a model in which the performance of symbolic domesticity supplanted devadasi practice and its range of emotional expression.

In this conjoining of revivalism and reform, Iyer paved the way for the establishment of the middle-class female dancer's subject position by replacing the participation of courtesan practitioners with his depiction of devadasi practice. Unlike the elite women who as they followed him onto the concert stage distanced themselves from devadasis, Iyer affiliated himself with the marginal legacy. Although he, along with other Music Academy officials, sponsored concerts by devadasis in the 1930s, his performance suggested that his impersonation could work as well as, if not better than, the "original."[11] This maneuver laid the groundwork for upper-caste women to replace devadasi practice with the revised concert form, claiming subject positions for themselves by representing and remaking courtesan practice. Iyer, and those who came to the urban stage after him, iconicized devadasis as emblems, not agents, of tradition.[12]

Once Iyer installed the devadasis' dance as a cultural symbol and acknowledged the need for its reform, Rukmini Devi refigured bharata natyam as a respectable accomplishment through which "women of good families" expressed cultural pride. Her project, like Iyer's, incorporated concerns of reform and revival but culminated more fully in the creation of the respectable-woman-as-dancer subject position. Her move to purify bharata natyam and especially her mitigation of sringara reinscribed the dance form with an impetus toward reform. Rukmini Devi injected choreography with those aspects most clearly associated with symbolic domesticity in the nationalist model: spirituality, nationalism, tradition, and sexual morality. However, these attributes of the "home" domain within the nationalist separation of spheres remained figurative: Devi's choreography and pedagogy enabled a move of "family women" into public spaces and into positions of authority in relation to the dance form. Moreover, a nascent (although Victorian) feminism and egalitarianism intertwined with her attention to gendered respectability (Meduri 1996: 331–36, 350–53; Srinivasan 1983). Through her preoccupation with respectability and her goal of purifying the form, Devi established a place for middle-class, upper-caste women on the resolutely public concert stage, negotiating but not fully resolving the questions around gender that the anti-nautch movement raised (Coorlawala 2005: 177).

Rukmini Devi entered the dance arena with a clear agenda: to eradicate the stigma on bharata natyam by removing its associations with courtesanship and to align it with national identity. In purifying the form, she responded to the anti-nautch movement's accusations of lasciviousness in dance performance. Although she rested the success of her project on the transfer of the dance practice to "women of quality," the mere "repopulation" of the dance (Allen 1997) did not suffice to secure bharata natyam's status. Rather, Rukmini Devi argued that the respectability of bharata natyam depended upon its shift to elite women and that its content required modification to suit these new practitioners. She mitigated the importance of sringara, maintaining that its explicit articulation was inappropriate for the middle-class girls and young women whom she taught at her Kalakshetra institution.[13] Overt eroticism, in her view, linked the dance form to devadasi lifestyles and therefore detracted from its spirituality, its classicism, and its ability to operate as a symbol of cultural pride. Devi's position accorded with that of the reform movements and, despite her pro-dance perspective, with some of the tenets of the anti-nautch campaign.

At the same time, Rukmini Devi also located in sadir an attenuated version of a once-glorious ancient tradition, a view that aligned her position with revivalism. She referenced a golden age for Indian performance in the period of classical Sanskrit, which, she maintained, offered respectable women artistic and other freedoms denied them in later years. As in nationalist discourse, the status of women equated here with civilizational merit. In Rukmini Devi's view, as in the revivalist-nationalist one, women's traditions represented a cultural authenticity removed from hybridizing colonial influences. Devi consolidated the subject position of the new practitioners by creating a historical narrative of respectability in which middle-class femininity supported the reconstruction of national culture.

Like the nineteenth-century nationalists, Rukmini Devi resolved the competing demands of reform and revival by giving elite women responsibility for protecting the classical traditions of indigenous culture. In mitigating the erotic and jocular components of sadir and highlighting religiosity and classicism, the new, respectable practitioner could move into increasingly public roles. Although Devi herself faced controversy when she gave her first public performance, the elements of symbolic domesticity—spirituality, classicism, and de-eroticized devotion—that she inserted into choreography, as well as her defense of its value, silenced her retractors. She did not fully answer questions raised by the dance's ability to embody both transgressive sexuality and an authentic cultural inheritance, but she countered aspersions cast on dance performance from orthodox quarters by foregrounding religion and tradition in choreography and pedagogy. Devi thus developed choreographic devices that signaled allegiance to a reformed tradition and provided middle-class women with an opportunity to move onto the concert stage without censure.

Rukmini Devi's dance dramas were one means through which she established symbolic domesticity in performance. Many of these works emphasize religious devotion cleansed of evident eroticism and highlight chaste love that culminates in matrimony. Several of these stories center on a female protagonist who, rather than lamenting her lover's neglect of her as in classical bhakti songs, adores a god or hero and eventually joins him in marriage. For example, Devi's *Kurma Avataram* (1974) portrays episodes from the Puranic creation story in which beings and objects arise from the churning of the cosmic ocean. One scenario depicts the emergence of Lakshmi, goddess of fortune, and her subsequent betrothal to Vishnu, maintainer of universal harmony.[14]

The scene begins with six male dancers ringing the front of the stage in a crescent shape. They stamp vigorously, kicking their feet up behind them and sinking into broad stances, cupping their hands loosely as if they held a rope. They reach toward a center point, throwing their torsos into the extension. They pull in unison away then rock back into their original stance as each sequence provides the momentum for the next extension.

A group of young women glides onto the stage. They lower their weight into a narrow, grounded stance while their feet flutter through a pulsative phrase. Appearing behind the men, they move toward center stage, two of the dancers holding a small curtain. The women drop the curtain and a beautifully attired female dancer appears, regal in her stillness. The attendants kneel before Lakshmi, their divine mistress. Lakshmi bursts into action with a sequence of virtuoso footwork, which her elegant arm positions echo. Her ladies-in-waiting emulate her expert rendition of the phrase, feet striking the floor, articulate fingers and arms adorning the staccato pattern.

After this brief interlude, a female dancer emerges from the wings and offers Lakshmi a flower garland. The lavishness of the flowers, as well as the care with which the handmaid carries it, suggests that this is the marriage garland with which Lakshmi will choose her spouse. When the men see her receive the garland, they present themselves for her polite, but discriminating consideration. Each male dancer wears a crown and jewelry, his attire as well as his bearing conveying his high birth. She barely gives them a passing glance, signaling her courteous rejection by directing the garland away from them. Again and again, Lakshmi changes course slightly, the uniformity of each turn revealing the constancy of her quest.

Finally, Vishnu enters the stage. His striking appearance and elegant demeanor win over the selective Lakshmi. She drapes the garland around his neck and retreats, bowing her head modestly and offering obeisance to her new husband. Vishnu joins her at center stage, encircling but not touching her shoulders as she bends her torso and lowers her weight so that she stands below him, tilting her head as though to rest it on his shoulder.[15] The ensemble encircles the couple, holding a canopy and parasol above them and depicting the scattering of flowers with their gestures, indicating their joy at this union.

This piece celebrates divine femininity by featuring Lakshmi, the most restrained and least independent of Hindu goddesses, and lauding both her companionate marriage and her reliant role in the new union. *Kurma Avataram* highlights the traits that Lakshmi shares with the bhadramahila: propriety, dignity, restriction to a conventional role within the patriarchal family, and a sexuality sublimated into domesticity, combined with confidence and volition in the outside world. In foregrounding a bhadramahila-like divine figure, the choreography offsets the nondomestic sexuality associated with dance practice. It defuses bharata natyam's potentially unsettling erotic idioms through a narrative that culminates in the domestication of the heroine's sexuality in marriage.

In Rukmini Devi's dance dramas generally, the shift of representational mode from first-person lyric to third-person narrative distances the performance from the erotic overtones of bhakti poetry. The bhakti model of personal expressions of longing and desire, when positioned alongside anti-nautch agitations, could cause the audience to conflate the dancer with the character she plays. The retention of sringara elements likewise appears to be a defense of the devadasi tradition. As indicated in chapter 1, the use of third-person narrative mitigates the expression of eroticism, because no character represents her emotion, and hence her desire, directly to the audience.

Kurma Avataram contributes to a gendered separation of spheres not only in its narrative, but also in its movement vocabulary. The male ensemble uses movement derived primarily from kathakali, a traditionally all-male dance drama form, while the female group performs bharata natyam movements. Accordingly, men's sequences emphasize wide positions, sharp, heavy gestures, and broad extensions, while the women's phrases deploy contained stances and a controlled, floating torso. The women's arm movements extend, but do not jut, out into space. The torso remains relatively still. Likewise, the female cast restricts abhinaya to delicate gestures of the hand and forearm and facial expressions, while the men use their full arms, torsos, and sometimes entire bodies in their portrayal of their characters. This delineation of female and male vocabularies suggests that women express dignity in curtailed behavior while men extend themselves out into the world. By contrasting male and female movement vocabularies, this dance drama bifurcates men's and women's conduct on a choreographic level, further consolidating the nationalist model of a parity and complementarity that depends upon difference.

Yet Rukmini Devi did not simply capitulate to a nationalist gendering of spheres. Rather, her valorization of domesticity legitimized her own public position as dancer, choreographer, and activist.[16] This approach enabled her not only to inhabit but also to refigure the public realm by claiming the role of innovator. The model that she established facilitated the entry of middle-class and upper-caste female dancers into public arenas of performance and choreography. Whereas male nationalists validated their claims to sovereignty through the refashioning of models of Indian womanhood, Rukmini Devi's interpretation of femininity allowed elite women to remake themselves.

One way that Devi introduced female self-fashioning to dance was through the invention of the role of dancer-choreographer.[17] At her Kalakshetra institution, Rukmini Devi provided middle-class women with positions of increased responsibility in dance, including instruction, choreography, and nattuvangam in addition to performance. Prior to the 1930s, dancers achieved renown as performers but generally did not take up choreography or instruction, especially in nritta. They also remained under the authority of a male guru. The latter trained the dancer, choreographed and arranged repertory items, and acted as nattuvanar, but he did not usually dance in public himself.

Rukmini Devi, by contrast, composed dance works and taught as well as performed; she also trained her students in music conducting,[18] eroding a gendered division of labor in which an individual could either be a dancer or a choreographer but not both. When she opened to middle-class women the positions of composer, instructor, and conductor, she initiated "the complete separation of [her] work from the traditional dance teachers" (in Sarada 1985: 50), which, for her, bolstered its respectability. The classed overtones of this shift dovetailed with the gendered ones: because middle-class women had themselves come to symbolize tradition and spirituality, their adoption of these positions imbued the dance form with a sense of increased classicism and reputability.

By creating occasions for dancers to learn to teach, choreograph, and conduct, she provided women with positions of authority in dance, offering them an informed, educated, and authoritative relationship to the choreography they performed. She gave her students opportunities for self-representation and for the representation of the form, which had been previously closed to the devadasi dancer. The shift extended to twentieth-century dancers the unique possibility of creating new work based on their own experiences as performers.[19] This gendered transformation then allowed the new choreographer-dancer to move from self-representation to interlocution for the tradition as a whole. Because this project constituted an authoritative middle-class feminine position through the exclusion of less "respectable" women, however, it met with resistance.

In contrast to Rukmini Devi, Balasaraswati insisted that the devadasi community provided bharata natyam with both its source and its continued artistic integrity. Whereas Rukmini Devi reformed, Balasaraswati defended, maintaining sringara's centrality to bharata natyam's aesthetics and religiosity. She argued that bharata natyam's successful melding of artistic and devotional agendas depended upon the cultivation of erotic sentiment and identified devadasis as the crucial link between sringara and bhakti. Sringara's compelling and complex nature, according to Balasaraswati, provided bharata natyam with ideal material for both dramatic expression and the cultivation of religious devotion through metaphor (Balasaraswati 1984: 15).

Balasaraswati's performance of *Samayamide*, a Telugu javali, portrays a contrasting image of femininity and sexuality to Rukmini Devi's *Kurma Avataram*.[20] This piece also celebrates Vishnu, but in his incarnation as the mischievous and amorous Krishna, rather than in his more imperious form as the preserver of universal stability—an inattentive lover rather than a magnanimous patriarch. The javali centers on the experiences of a female protagonist but differs from the

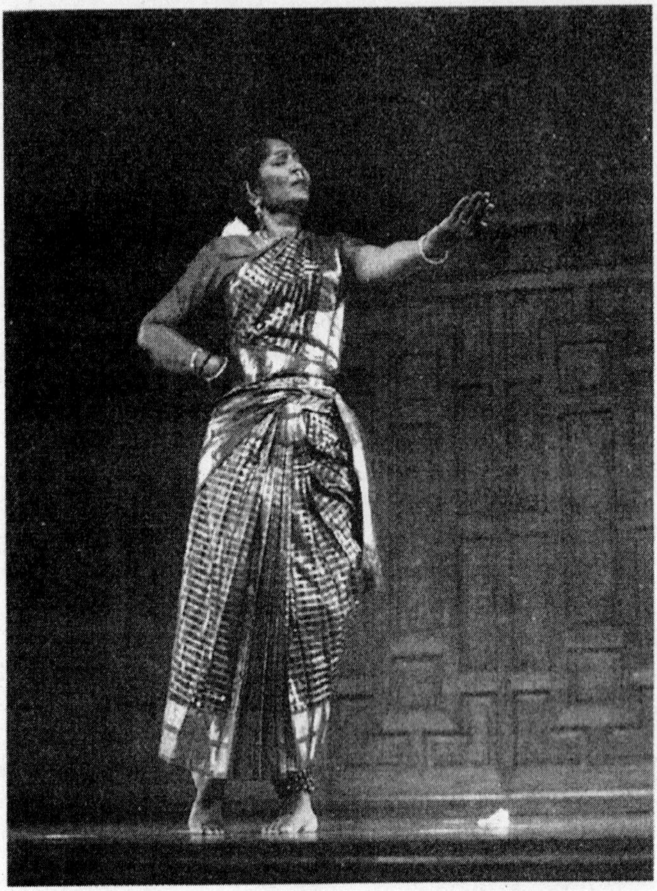

Figure 15: Balasaraswati's nayika offers a sarcastic rejoinder to a perfidious lover. © Jan Steward 1986.

dance drama by foregrounding her extradomestic sexual desire and linking it to devotional passion. Although Balasaraswati also performed pieces that expressed a more distant, overtly respectful piety, her interpretation of items such as *Samayamide Javali* exemplified her defense of sringara through concerns of gender, class, and sexuality.

The piece opens with a dancer emerging from the wings as the musicians conclude their *alapana*, or musical introduction. She pauses at center stage as the singer delivers the first lines of the song: "This is the moment, my lord. Come [to me]; do not delay." The dancer renders the song in mudras, first beginning with a literal translation of the text. Thumb and forefinger meet and then separate to indicate "an instant" while a hand rotates and fingers tip toward the ground to signal "this." She rests her palm at her chest, indicating "my," while her thumb raised above a closed fist denotes "man." Her forefinger and thumb, joined at their extended tips, trace a vertical line in front of her body, suggesting the passing of time, while a single flat palm, facing outward with a slight wave places the previous concept in the negative: do not delay. The dancer then launches the sanchari bhavas, which expand upon the literal rendition to invoke poetic tropes and develop the tone of the piece. Images such as "lotus-eyed one" indicate her admiration; when the dancer extends her arm and grasps her own wrist as if it were Krishna's, she signals the heroine's anxiety.

The section that follows reveals to the audience the illicit nature of the character's love. The dancer rests the tips of a thumb and forefinger at the base of her neck, while her other arm ends in a fist with thumb raised, the combination denoting "husband." A flat palm draws a horizontal line, suggesting "[this] place," while another flat palm in front of the body signals "no"; the whole phrase means "my husband is not here." An articulate hand traces the upper lip, the line of a mustache referring to an older man—the character's father-in-law—who, she tells us, also has no reason to return here. The dancer then introduces an element of sarcasm to her hitherto loving monologue by referring to Krishna's numerous liaisons. She portrays his inattention by extending her arm vertically, conjoining a wave of the hand with an indifferent look in the opposite direction, and queries this neglect in light of his amorous exploits with others.

In the final section, the dramatic frame broadens when the heroine acknowledges that their initial union occurred only in a dream. A revelation that the object of her desire is none other than Vishnu, Lord of the Universe himself, follows. The juxtaposition of the character's intimate emotion with the impersonal nobility of the god comes across in her penultimate gestures: palm opening to indicate "flower," followed by hands gently tracing the eyes, she once again refers to him in the term of affection—"lotus-eyed one"—used earlier in the piece. The dancer then assumes one of Vishnu's characteristic full-body iconographic poses, right foot crossed over left, elbows lifted with wrists flexed, palms open, and ring finger bent away from the other extended fingers.

This piece follows a typical bhakti pattern, wherein a song expresses devotion through a young heroine's love for an absent god-hero.[21] Because the anti-nautch campaign had blamed the "wanton" lifestyle of the devadasis on the "lewdness" of the dance and vice versa, a defense of sringara in the early to mid-twentieth century implied a defense of the devadasi system. Although sringara bhakti pieces articulate sexual desire through the words of young, elite heroines, when performed in the revival and post-revival periods they reminded dancers and audience members of the courtesan lifestyle of devadasi practitioners. Although most viewers recognized the tropes of bhakti literature, reformist discourse would have colored their reception of erotic references in dance so that sringara also echoed devadasi mores. Balasaraswati's defense of sringara, then, upheld not only the tropes of devadasi performance practice, but also the authority of the devadasi community, refuting a seemingly inevitable replacement of devadasi dancers by upper-caste performers.

In advocating for the devadasi legacy, Balasaraswati, like anti-nautch reformers, conflated dramatic representation and community associations but reversed the valuation placed on these components. Instead of seeing the interconnections between sringara bhakti and the devadasi community as inviting reform, she presented sringara bhakti as emblematic of the dance tradition's greatness. As a plea for the preservation of indigenous practices in light of reformist demands, her strategy on one level matched that of nineteenth-century revivalists. She diverged from nationalist-revivalists, however, by using this recourse to the past and the accompanying gendering of tradition in order to defend marginal, lower-caste women and their artistic practice rather than to exculpate orthodox, indigenous patriarchy. This model allowed her to inscribe a subject position through which she, as a devadasi, represented a hereditary practice and contested the replacement of the devadasis by elite women. Within her conservatism lay a resistance to the reform of bharata natyam as well as to the classed assumption of authority on which that refiguration depended.

This strategy of revivalism with a difference intertwined traditional representations of gender behavior with a valorization of indigenous, precolonial models of independent womanhood. It anticipated a late-twentieth-century debate over the gender politics of bhakti. Beginning in the 1980s, dancers critiqued bhakti from an overtly feminist point of view, challenging the premise that the pining female protagonist symbolizes a devotee who stands helpless before a never fully attentive god. Feminist performers maintained that by representing the worshipper as a devoted young woman and the god as her philandering lover, bhakti poetry reinscribes a sexual double standard on the human level and reinforces gender discrimination by treating a heterosexual love as emblematic of the inherently unequal human-divine relationship.[22]

However, because the bhakti movement offered a level of increased freedom to specific women, Indian feminist authors, such as Uma Chakravarti (1989), Veena Talwar Oldenburg (1991), and Amrit Srinivasan (1987), looked at bhakti from another angle, investigating the religious movement and its artistic products as a model of precolonial social critique. They focused not on the gender imbalances of the poetry but on the autonomy, however incomplete, that the lifestyle of female bhakti poets and of courtesans who performed devotional songs and dances allowed. These writers sought out paradigms of precolonial egalitarianism in order to challenge the conservative patriarchal idea that India inherited feminism from the West.[23]

These feminist authors relied upon revivalist discourse by demonstrating parallels to European post-Enlightenment values in indigenous practices. At the same time, they reconstructed this past differently. Revivalist movements, although they internalized colonial critiques, remained conservative as they sought to preserve the status quo, defending indigenous patriarchy and class hierarchy by valorizing the "protections" that tradition offered to "vulnerable" members of society (Sangari 1989). By contrast, anticolonial feminist reconstructions used precolonial models of equality and resistance to interrogate the inequities of Indian society. They strove to dismantle social hierarchies while also challenging a supposedly determinative link between feminism and colonialism.

Balasaraswati anticipated this strategy of revivalism through difference by deploying precolonial practices as a form of class critique and by positioning models of female volition and (partial) autonomy in indigenous practices. Although her strategies parallel the anticolonial feminist use of indigenous models for egalitarian agendas, Balasaraswati's approach was not an activist one. In addition, her resistance to an upper-caste assumption of power within the dance form rested upon an idealized, sophisticated devadasi subject and therefore obscured the extent to which devadasis were subject to gender oppression. Balasaraswati resisted the erosion of devadasi preeminence in dance and defended traditional protocol primarily as a criticism of caste-based appropriation, not of gender subordination. Her celebration of sringara defended hereditary praxis through a class critique in which gender underlined concerns of community authority and aesthetic efficacy.

This maneuver did, however, restore a partial authority to the devadasi community to influence the present and future of bharata natyam. By valorizing the precedent set by a community of marginal practitioners, Balasaraswati posited a different gender problematic from that of nationalist practitioners such as Iyer and Devi, reinscribing devadasi practice as a site of agency. The thematic, however, remained similar to that of the dance reformers: she consolidated subjectivity and authority through the representation of gender.[24]

Balasaraswati's strategies, like those of Iyer and Devi, indicate that from nineteenth- and early-twentieth-century reform and revival campaigns bharata natyam acquired the ability to represent and query existing gender discourses. Moreover, gender concerns in bharata natyam underlined other categories of identity, such as class, caste, and national affiliations, alongside individual subjectivity. Early-twentieth-century practitioners grappled with reformist and revivalist agendas, reinstalling, rather than resolving, the "women's question" in choreography and in debates around dance. The competing perspectives of revival-era dancers indicate not only that the "women's question" remained incompletely resolved in bharata natyam but also that it endured because, for twentieth-century dancers, it remained highly productive for subject constitution. It therefore set the stage for a subsequent reworking of gender discourses and subjectivity in the late twentieth century.

Subjects and Their Others in Late-Twentieth-Century Bharata Natyam

Late-twentieth-century performers continued to examine the issues raised in the revival, addressing their own position as public figures and examining the suitability of explicit sringara references in choreography. They likewise considered the significance of the devadasi tradition, usually defending it rather than critiquing it overtly. Through these discussions, they legitimized their own practice of the form. However, dancers of the 1980s and 1990s also engaged more explicitly with international representations of Indian women. As in the case of early-twentieth-century choreography, dancers deployed reformist and revivalist discourses, responding, in the process, to (neo-)colonial interpretations of women's status in India. Like performers at the end of the colonial period, late-twentieth-century practitioners confronted representations of Indian women as both objects of oppression and symbols of a great tradition.

Despite the demise of imperial rule in India, neocolonial accounts of atrocities against Indian women continue to link gender subjugation to an atavistic abasement of Indian society in general. As Uma Narayan (1997) argues, international attention to Indian women reveals its colonial underpinnings by emphasizing the degrading effects of culture and tradition; it does not attend to either systemic oppression or individual acts of exploitation. Journalistic, popular, and scholarly representations identify the suffering of Indian women as a product of repressive customs rather than in the actions of particular individuals with contemporary, material motives.[25]

The positioning of gender oppression elsewhere, among marginal communities, is not limited to Western accounts. Rather, as Anannya Bhattacharjee (1992) indicates in her discussion of emigrant Indians and their perceptions of domestic violence, a middle-class public reinforces its own universalized position by naming and identifying the oppressive practices of "others." According to Bhattacharjee, the nonresident Indian bourgeoisie participates in this "exnomination" (Bhattacharjee 1992) by locating gender subjugation at the margins of society; they therefore avoid interrogating their own sexist assumptions. Such a process creates alterity as much as it represents it. This understanding of gender subjugation, Bhattacharjee maintains, allows a middle-class, diasporic public to leave their own oppressive behavior unexamined and to reinstall themselves as the interlocutor for the subjugation of "others."

Adherents to religious orthodoxy and other defenders of indigenous patriarchy have used the colonial/reform interface to criticize feminists and other politically active women as imitators of "the West."[26] A late-twentieth-century rise in religious fundamentalism, both in India and globally, created ample opportunity for conservatives to level this critique: fundamentalists defended "local" cultures and religious practices, selectively identifying what foreign elements needed to be purged and what could be retained. Thus, in the case of India, Hindu fundamentalists berated feminists (and other progressives) as, in Parama Roy's terms, "inadequate substitutes" for "the real thing (Indianness, femininity)" (1998: 129) and as "Westernized elites" who were out of touch with the populace as a whole (Nandy, in Rajan 1993: 17).

This conflation of activism with Westernization added to the double bind that the late-twentieth-century bharata natyam dancer faced. On the one hand, dancers contended with a practice that emerged from the collision of gendered reform and revival debates and inherited a responsibility to represent an empowered, yet respectable, Indian womanhood. Because of the continual criticism leveled at India for its treatment of women, the lower castes, and minorities, colonial and neocolonial accounts identified "women's issues" as arenas for reform. On the other hand, given the fundamentalist dismissal of progressive social movements, a dancer who embraces politics too overtly runs the risk of losing widespread acceptance or even, as in the case of Mallika Sarabhai, punishment by the state.[27] Many dancers who address gender issues find ways of integrating the representation of women into a celebration or at least acknowledgment of the merits of "Indian tradition." Ex-nomination becomes a device for raising gender critiques without jeopardizing audience support.

When bharata natyam dancers present their work internationally, they confront two habits of ex-nomination, each of which positions them differently. A mainstream Western viewing public treats the dancer, as a South Asian woman and/or as a representative of Indian traditions, as its other. Among elite Indians and Indian emigrants, by contrast, the dancer operates as subject through a class-based ex-nomination that positions alterity among the poorer classes, within lower castes, and in villages. The middle-class Indian female dancer, then, in an international context, is simultaneously both self/subject and an other. I suggest in the following pages that late-twentieth-century dancers grapple with competing pressures: a neocolonial, popular perspective that positions them as oppressed and silenced Indian women, and a habit of ex-nomination in their own communities and in those they engage with internationally that casts them as an interlocutor for others. Reformist and revivalist discourses endure in choreography because they provide avenues for dancers to install themselves as subjects and to represent those marginal to the dance milieu.

Late-twentieth-century performers rely on the work of the revival by deploying colonial and nationalist gender ideology as they address dominant representations of Indian women. This international outlook acquires significance whether the specific work of choreography circulates globally or not as the discourses that dancers engage with become consistently more transnational, through the representation of India and its social concerns, and as Indian cities themselves become increasingly globalized. Choreographers continue to rely on the solutions provided to the "women's question" in the early twentieth century, celebrating the virtues and strengths of the women of India's past and identifying gender oppression in the experience of women who cannot represent themselves. They continue a model wherein dancers install their own subject position by speaking for their others. In the late twentieth century, the other to the "respectable woman" is less likely to be a devadasi and more likely to be a woman from another time period or location. Late-twentieth-century performers thus relied on the strategies of the revival while also refiguring them, inscribing their own subject positions into the dance not only by representing the dance tradition, as in the revival, but also by speaking for those excluded from the public arts sphere.

Chitra Visweswaran's *Stree Shakti* (The Power of Woman, or Woman Goddess [1995])[28]—depicts iconic female characters from the canon of the Hindu epics. Using the vocabulary of classical bharata natyam, Visweswaran, the sole performer, narrates a central event in the life of each heroine, foregrounding both the character's volition and her devotion to her family and society. Visweswaran portrays Sita, heroine of the *Ramayana*, through the (in)famous "chastity test" that the goddess undergoes at the insistence of her husband Rama. The epic places Sita in a central but not active role: its events unfold because of her abduction by the demon-king Ravana. Although Sita lives in the demon-lord's home, she rejects his advances and remains faithful to Rama. She is so dedicated to her husband that she even refuses rescue by Hanuman, the monkey-god who is Rama's second-in-command, because such a deliverance would entail touching a male other than her spouse. In spite of Sita's unwavering fidelity, Rama, upon defeating Ravana in battle, rejects his wife, treating her with disdain until she proves her virtue by entering a burning pyre and emerging unharmed.[29]

Foregrounding Sita's resilience to the humiliation that Rama inflicts upon her, *Stree Shakti* depicts the goddess's entrance into the assembly formed by Rama at the time of his victory. Visweswaran emerges from an upstage side wing. Her diagonally placed foot tilts her weight off center so that her body tips into a delicate curve. Her outer arm circles her face and her articulate fingers tip toward her chin. The mudra and the dancer's averted gaze suggest that, out of modesty, Sita has veiled herself. Her feet begin a strong but narrow stamping pattern, one foot chasing the other as she traverses the stage. With her head turned aside and her gaze lowered, Sita exhibits discomfort with appearing in public while her radiant expression indicates her eagerness and joy at her impending reunion with Rama.

When she reaches center stage, she turns, wide-eyed and beaming, extending her arms in expectation of reconciliation. Sita addresses Rama, offering herself to his protection and humbly indicating her gratitude at her rescue. The expression turns to one of dismay, however, when Rama rejects her. Wringing her hands in a plea, Sita promises that she has been true to him. Chin dropping, this time out of dejection, not modesty, Sita retreats from her beloved.

Visweswaran assumes Rama's role momentarily when, with lifted chest and raised chin, she extends her arm, sending Sita away. Eyes flashing with anger, she indicates Rama's dismissal of his wife. This response prompts Sita to enter a burning pyre in order to confirm her virtue. Her shimmering hands trace multiple trajectories, diagonals and verticals crossing one another to demonstrate the height of the conflagration and the breadth of the pyre. Her bulging eyes and fearsome expression demonstrate the ferocity of the flames. Her hands cease their furious movement and her demeanor shifts: she appears dignified and radiant in her resolve. Hands meeting at her chest, Sita entreats Agni, the god of fire, to authenticate her assertion. She enters the fire and, having calmly endured its heat, reemerges unharmed.

Stree Shakti celebrates Hindu divine femininity and lauds valiant figures from a mythological past. At the same time, it emphasizes female sacrifice and reinscribes the feminine principle into the domestic sphere, depicting, for example, Sita's strength through her devotion to her spouse. Visweswaran describes the piece as her "answer to feminism," identifying it as a response to the androgyny that, she suggests, feminism promotes (personal correspondence 1999). She maintains that the work preserves sex difference and validates the feminine domain by celebrating the strength of women in epic literature. She contrasts this depiction of Indian women with sensationalist accounts of gender oppression in India such as the BBC's coverage of dowry deaths (personal correspondence 1999). This piece addresses the colonialist underpinnings of much (global) gender discourse as it portrays Indian women. It echoes revivalist discourses by self-consciously proclaiming the strength of Indian womanhood in response to Western/global representations of Indian women as iconically degraded, suggesting that India's heroic women do not need the pity of the West.[30] As such, the work refutes neocolonial censure by extolling the virtues of India's past, through which women enjoyed freedoms but remained loyal to their homes, families, and societies.

Stree Shakti relies upon the bhadramahila figure by foregrounding Sita's volition alongside her devotion to her spouse. The work fuses narrative and movement vocabulary, (re-)inscribing feminine respectability into bharata natyam. Visweswaran's celebration of a divine bhadramahila depicts Indian women as symbols not of abjection but of domesticated power. Especially as the piece circulates internationally, it counters the racist assumptions of much Western thought, both conventional and feminist, that Indian women require rescue from their oppressive traditions (Mohanty 1984; Spivak 1988). In foregrounding the virtue of feminine volition and sacrifice, Visweswaran puts forth an idealized feminine subject position that counters neoimperialist stereotypes of Indian women. As in the case of Rukmini Devi, such celebrations of the status quo allow a choreographer to legitimize her own status as a public figure. *Stree Shakti*, despite its late-twentieth-century production, relies upon the "remaking" of Indian women (Roy 1998: 129) that enabled bharata natyam's transition to the concert stage in the 1930s.

Where *Stree Shakti* lauds orthodox Hindu ideals of femininity as signs of power rather than of submission, Y. G. Madhuvanthy's *Kanya* (1991) reveals the enduring oppression that some Indian women face in daily life.[31] *Kanya*—meaning girl or maiden—tackles gender issues in a dance drama format that deploys bharata natyam–derived choreography. Madhuvanty raises similar concerns to those addressed in the nineteenth-century reform movements, such as female education and the detrimental effects of child marriage. The piece also adds a contemporary problem to reformist concerns by introducing dowry murder as another example of the oppression of women.

The work opens with the main character, Meena, as a small child, playing with her brother in a village. Their camaraderie and equality ends when two adult dancers—Meena's parents—separate the two siblings. They offer Meena's brother books and send him to school, keeping their daughter home to learn domestic tasks. When her brother returns from school, Meena notices that he neglects his texts in favor of play, and she uses her spare moments to consult his books. She teaches herself arithmetic, practicing on foodstuffs and household items, which she lines up on the floor. Her gesturing index finger marks her counting as she leans over the tabulations, utterly engrossed.

Meena's fate changes when she notes a sudden decrease in the number of objects. She leaps to her feet to sound the alarm that someone has stolen her family's property. After the town's denizens apprehend the thief, Meena demonstrates her system and her community realizes that her mathematical skill saved their resources. Her parents acknowledge her talents and send her to school with her brother, allowing her to continue her education into adolescence.

Meena's childhood playmates are not so fortunate. Two of her friends leave the village for marriage. Celebration attends the wedding of the first friend. Meena, now played by an adolescent dancer, circulates through a crowded stage filled with lavish ornamentation and elegantly attired guests. Despite this happy beginning, disaster strikes when the friend's husband, barely more than a stranger to her, dies. The girl, now a widow, must live a life of strict asceticism, rendered practically a servant in her marital home.

The family of the second friend ushers her away quickly, with little ceremony, foreshadowing an even worse fate than that of youthful widowhood. Meena pines over her missing friend, but this anxiety doesn't compare with her shock when she receives news of the friend's mistreatment at the hands of her affinal family. The in-laws are attempting to generate a larger dowry by threatening the girl. The final blow comes in a letter. Meena opens the message and her facial expression twists from the now-accustomed sadness into horror: her friend has died at the hands of her in-laws.

The second act commences on a brighter note as the adult Meena leaves her village to pursue further education. Her move into middle-class life provides its own tribulations, albeit more minor ones. She arrives in the city (the location conveyed by a backdrop of tall buildings and a sound-score of traffic noise) alone and frightened, eyes darting from one side to another. She places her hands at her mouth, signaling her fear, and extends them in disorientation. Meena contends with the crush of city life, miming collisions with other pedestrians and objects. Her panic eventually subsides, and she acclimates to the city. She trains in Carnatic music, seated cross-legged on the floor, clapping in time to a basic music lesson, and rendering elementary vocal exercises. As a recorded voice calls out *solkattu*, spoken rhythmic syllables, Meena performs rudimentary bharata natyam exercises. Bharata natyam, an avocation for Meena, endorses her new status as an urban, middle-class woman.

The dance drama takes a reformist approach to gender issues, concerning itself with the oppression of Indian (village) women. Despite its portrayal of gender subordination, however, *Kanya*'s women do not merely function as "the ground of the discourse" (Mani 1990: 117). The piece foregrounds a main character who refigures her own position through cultural as well as professional accomplishments. Meena, educated and employed, establishes her subject position and acts as interlocutor for the women silenced by their oppression, the child widow and the murdered bride.

By acquiring mastery over the markers of both symbolic domesticity and pubic achievement, Meena installs herself as a respectable modern woman. In presenting subjugation as a framing device to Meena's triumph over her circumstances, the piece reinstates the nationalist resolution of the women's question by suggesting that Meena corrects these wrongs not through activism or agitation for systemic change, but by becoming a role model for other village women. Here, the nationalist gender paradigm offers class mobility to one of the bhadramahila's others. *Kanya* unfixes a class-gender configuration through the protagonist's transformation from marginalized villager to modern woman.

For *Kanya*'s Chennai-based audience, however, this narrative of obstacles surmounted remains more vexed. Although the character crosses a boundary between the represented and the interlocutor, the urban viewer's subject position goes untroubled. The alterity of rural areas in comparison to urban centers such as Chennai allows viewers to embrace present-day reform discourses without questioning their own practices, values, and assumptions. Instead, an urban viewership can project its assessment of gender issues onto the culturally and geographically distant village. Spectators can then continue to identify gender oppression as occurring elsewhere.

Mallika Sarabhai's *In Search of Devi* (1999) takes a more critical approach to the representation of women than either *Stree Shakti* or *Kanya*. Sarabhai turns a reformist lens on the heroines of the Sanskrit epics and mythology, the subjects invoked in revivalist discourse. Sarabhai retells stories of the eminent women of classical literature, locating female agency in some episodes and using others to illustrate the subjugation of women. On the one hand, these sketches subvert revivalist maneuvers by attending to the persecution of the very heroines that orthodox discourse glorifies. On the other hand, the work, like *Kanya*, still allows

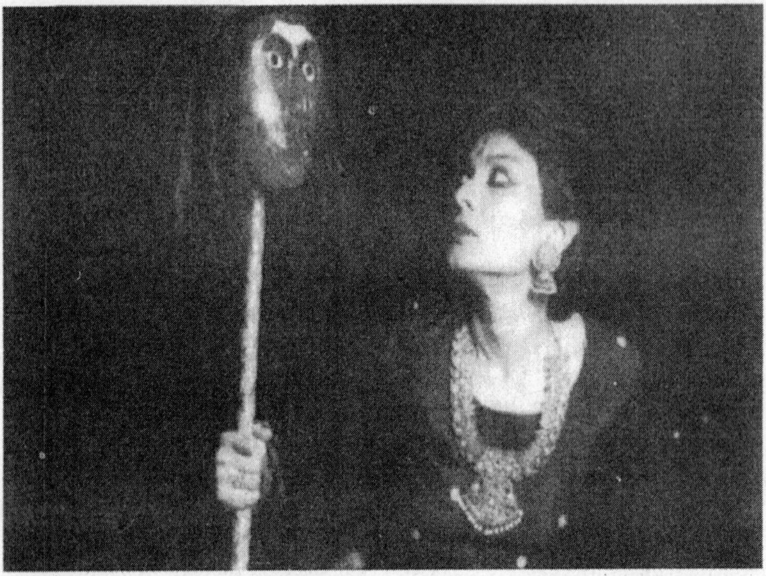

Figure 16: Mallika Sarabhai in *In Search of Devi*. Courtesy of Darpana Academy of Performing Arts, Ahmedabad, India.

its audience a level of ex-nomination by situating gender oppression elsewhere, among women of a mythological past.

The piece opens as Sarabhai, the sole performer, briskly enters the stage. Her cropped hair and tailored silk trousers juxtaposed with stage makeup and temple-style jewelry signal that a revisionist version of classical Indian dance will follow. Sarabhai installs herself as, literally, a speaking subject when she launches into a series of scenes that combine English-language prose monologues, the dramatic techniques of European and Indian theater forms, and the movement vocabulary of bharata natyam and kuchipudi.

Although most of the sketches portray the subjugation of the heroines of canonical Hindu literature, Sarabhai's retelling of the Puranic story of Savitri and Satyavan highlights a woman's volition. Sarabhai plays Savitri, a young wife, representing the other characters—her husband, Satyavan, and Yama, the god of death—through the manipulation of a stylized mask. Savitri first appears sitting under a tree, the couple's happiness apparent in their affectionate position: the mask rests in Savitri's lap as though Satyavan is reclining as his wife embraces him. Satyavan's death scene echoes the same shape, reinforcing the poignancy of Savitri's loss as she cradles the mask in her arms. Satyavan's unexpected demise devastates his adoring spouse; her body tension and her thrown-back head articulate her anguish.

Rather than simply succumb to a life of widowhood, however, Savitri follows her husband to the underworld and confronts Yama, the god of death. Extending the mask at arm's length, she repeatedly appeals to Yama to restore her spouse to her. The underworld becomes increasingly terrifying, but Savitri continues to give chase. Finally, Yama, both exasperated and impressed, acknowledges Savitri's bravery and devotion, offering to fulfill a wish of Savitri's if she gives up her quest. Savitri asks for a boon of one hundred sons. When Yama grants it, she points out his mistake: since he himself had commended her chastity, he must know that she could not have sons without her husband. Her triumphant tone and sharp, clear movements proclaim her success in this contest of wits. Yama, acknowledging his defeat, restores Satyavan to life and Savitri leaves victorious.

Sarabhai shifts to a first-person commentary from Savitri's point of view on the story and its use in the glorification of female self-sacrifice. Using the term *sati*—literally, "good woman"—and playing on the expected use of the term, Sarabhai disentangles the orthodox conflation of a virtuous woman with a woman who ends her life. Sarabhai tells her audience that Savitri is a sati, a good woman, not because she followed her husband into death but because she showed fortitude, intelligence, and skill. She concludes with the statement that "I [Savitri] am a sati mostly because I won." Sarabhai thereby supplants the expected meaning of sati, a woman who relinquishes her life, with an alternate definition of a good woman as a brave, resourceful, and successful one.

This piece, by valorizing a sati who lives, deconstructs both revivalist and reformist discourse on widow immolation, in which women who die either embody a heroic devotion to duty or symbolize an abject element of society in need of rescue.[32] A conservative, revivalist interpretation of the Savitri story emphasizes her willingness to relinquish her own life when she accompanies her husband into death. Savitri can be portrayed as a sati in two senses. First, she is a good woman who demonstrates her unwavering loyalty to her husband and refuses the possibility of remarriage or any kind of sexual life as a widow. Second, she also appears to be a woman who is willing to die in the interest of this devotion, determined to follow her husband into the afterlife. As such, she demonstrates, in Rajan's terms, the sati's ascribed "exceptionality" in facing death without fear or pain (1993: 20–21).

In a reformist interpretation, by contrast, Savitri's sacrifice exemplifies the subjugation of women within Indian traditions. Here, the widow who dies emerges as the quintessential victim, a woman oppressed not simply by men but by culture and tradition. The sati appeared in colonial discourse, for example, as a woman who required rescue and whose existence justified imperial intervention (Spivak 1988: 297). Depending on their point of view, reformers treat the sati as either symbolic of the barbaric nature of Indian society or emblematic of the universal oppression of women, which takes its worst form in the customs of the third world (Leslie 1992; Mani 1990; Spivak 1988).

The site of the performance amplifies the interrogation of both revivalist and reformist perspectives on Indian women. The piece opened a show on goddesses in Indian art at the Smithsonian Museum's Sackler Gallery in Washington, D.C. Sarabhai's performance challenges revivalist interpretations of the collection by querying the assumption that goddess worship necessarily accords women any degree of autonomy.[33] By emphasizing a heroic female character who survives and whose journey to the netherworld serves a positive purpose, Sarabhai finds a way out of, in Gayatri Spivak's terms, the double bind of subject versus object formulation.[34] At the same time, however, the appearance of themes drawn from reformist and revivalist movements indicates the extent to which even this explicitly feminist piece struggles to break out of, and provide alternatives to, colonialist and nationalist discursive frames.

In the Savitri excerpt, Sarabhai addresses a Washington, D.C. audience that is familiar with the campaigns against sati and distant from actual instances of widow immolation. The piece therefore evokes oppressive actions that its viewers already know about and presumably oppose but intervenes less directly into the immediate experience of its urban, middle-class, predominately Indian expatriate audience. Thus, like *Kanya*, this sketch breaks down a boundary between the represented and the representer but also permits a level of ex-nomination on the part of its audience. The work interrogates the promotion of the goddess exhibit it opened but confronts its viewers' potentially oppressive practices indirectly rather than posing an overt challenge to spectators' unexamined gender assumptions.

Visweswaran, Madhuvanty, and Sarabhai all tackle questions of gender equality and subjugation more explicitly than the practitioners of the revival did. Each of their choreographies queries representations of Indian womanhood self-consciously and with a marked intentionality. At the same time, all continue to deploy discourses of reform and revival. While Visweswaran celebrates iconic women, Madhuvanty and Sarabhai point to enduring inequalities. Each of these choreographers takes a position on dominant discourses on gender while retaining the early-twentieth-century problematic of installing subjectivity through the representation of other women.

Unable to Remember Roop Kanwar: Subjectivity, Representation, and Resistance

The choreographer and scholar Ananya Chatterjea's *Unable to Remember Roop Kanwar* (1997) questions the very possibility of representing gender oppression and widow immolation in particular. The piece addresses the problem, for anti-colonial feminists, posed by neoimperialist and religious fundamentalist representations of agency and subjectivity. Whereas Sarabhai's work replaces a practice that viewers can agree to oppose with a portrayal of female volition, Chatterjea's choreography tackles the quandary that a nearly contemporary instance of widow immolation presents for an investigation of subjectivity and gender.

In 1987, eighteen-year-old Roop Kanwar died on her husband's funeral pyre in Deorala, a village in Rajasthan. The death represented an isolated and unresolved instance of suicide or murder that generated a reaction that overshadowed the actual immolation itself (Rajan 1993: 16; Hawley 1994: 6–11). Kanwar's demise sparked a proliferation of commemorations of female self-sacrifice. Indian feminists mobilized against the death and its valorization, while conservative forces rallied in its favor. Representatives of orthodox Hinduism as well as wealthy elites of rural Rajasthani communities celebrated the sati as an emblem of Hindu feminine devotion and of Rajasthani heroism. The Indian government, although slow to prosecute those who initiated or abetted the immolation, instituted new regulations against the glorification of sati (Rajan 1993: 16–17). The international press responded with sensationalized accounts of the subjugation of third-world women. This instance of gender oppression signaled, for some international commentators, India's ostensible proclivity toward the subjugation of women as well as toward religious extremism.

This sati, as a traditionalized, spectacularized form of gender oppression, reactivated reformist and revivalist discourses in which women appear either as victims in need of rescue or as brave women who go willingly to their deaths. Revivalist and reformist discourses reemerged in the Kanwar case in which the dead woman shifted from an individual into an iconicized representation of either heroic sacrifice or of women's universal subjugation. This incident, by bringing these enduring protectionist and laudatory discourses to the fore, posed a "methodological crisis" for Indian feminists and feminist theory (Rajan 1993: 19). Feminists agitating against the celebration of Kanwar's death struggled to distance themselves from both the patriarchal defense of Hindu orthodoxy and the neocolonial sensationalism of accounts of gender oppression in India. Activists and authors such as Kumkum Sangari (1987) qualified arguments that hinged on individual volition through attention to the mistreatment of widows in conservative sectors of Hindu society. Feminists likewise highlighted the imperialist underpinnings of international feminist criticism of the status of Indian women and the antifeminist nature of discourses of protection that referenced the abjection of Indian women.

Chatterjea's *Unable to Remember Roop Kanwar*, a work for four performers, tackles this dilemma directly. The piece opens on a darkened stage with a voice-over monologue projected over the sound system. The speaker explains Kanwar's immolation and the reaction it generated. The lights come up gradually to create a pool of red-illumined space into which a solo dancer, clad in an orange and red cotton sari, crawls. The vibrancy of her attire contrasts with her tentative creeping and her frantic glances from side to side. Meanwhile, the voice-over describes the debate over volition that Kanwar's death provoked and reminds the audience

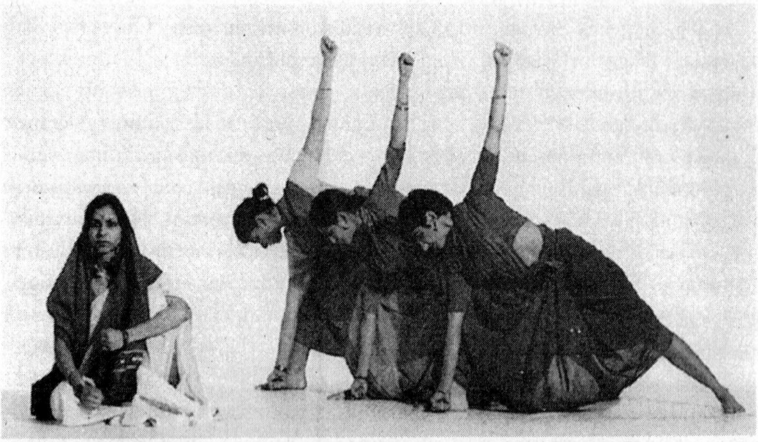

Figure 17: Rashmi Singh, Veeti Tandon, Ananya Chatterjea, and Aditi Dhruv in Ananya Chatterjea's *Unable to Remember Roop Kanwar.* Photograph by Erik Saulitis.

that "this focus on subjectivity is not new to Indian politics." The dancer rotates onto her back with a terrified expression and scuttles away from a source of fear invisible to the audience.

The dancer reaches up and claws her hands while arching her back and bending her knees. As the speaker describes British colonial accounts of the sati's pain, the dancer's body relaxes momentarily, although her face still conveys anguish. The disembodied voice comments on the hypocrisy of the colonial critique: "The British used these 'facts' to berate Indian villagers for their barbarity; never mind the women burned at the stake as witches at home." The dancer rolls over onto her bent knees and faces down, with her arms outstretched. She pauses and lifts her head.

The narrator explains: "When we started to create the piece, we tried to remember Roop Kanwar." The dancer, still prone, runs her hands along her arms as if trying to remove something, then lifts herself onto all fours and edges her way across the floor. The voice goes on to comment that "we also did not want to remember and objectify her like the colonial and media accounts did" as the dancer extends her arms along the floor. She drags her lower body as she heads toward the wings while the voice explains that the company does not claim to represent the sati but instead chose to treat widow immolation as part of the global phenomenon of domestic violence. The narrator tells the audience that the dancers want to remember resistance, commemorating not those women who die but those who risk their lives to struggle against subjugation. The relator becomes more impassioned as she gives examples of oppression, each followed by a refrain of "we say no." The solo dancer backs offstage and the lights lower until the narrator's "no" carries across the darkness.

The lights come up to illuminate a cross-section of the stage, which, awash in hard white, contrasts with the fiery hue of the previous section. A lone woman enters dressed in a cotton sari and dragging a long, patterned cloth behind her. She sits cross-legged and sings as she mimes the performance of domestic tasks while a trio of dancers casts long shadows behind her. The dancers traverse the stage, following one another in a pattern that alternates between running, stamping, and crouching. The ensemble exits, and the soloist rises to wrap herself in her shawl. Her facial expression remains calm and composed until she realizes that other lengths of cloth follow the first. The fabric overwhelms her; she becomes entangled, struggles, and comes to a halt with the wrap covering her entire body, including her face.

A sole performer walks out on stage wearing a red veil interwoven with a gold thread, reminiscent of a Rajasthani bridal shawl.[35] She staggers and weaves as she traverses the stage. Suddenly, she stops and walks with determination. She falls backward slightly and resumes her rocking walk, arms raised as if in a state of ecstasy, while her legs wobble underneath her.

An amplified voice interrupts the silence of the somnambulant solo. The offstage narrator recites a poem on dowry-related violence, beginning with the onomatopoetic "Whack!" Two dancers appear onstage, unseen by the swaying soloist, and, in conjunction with a second exclamation, jump in place with arched backs and bent legs. As the poem recounts the cruelty a new bride encountered at the hands of her husband and in-laws, the dancers stamp in bent-leg positions, their articulate footwork reminiscent of bharata natyam and odissi. They straighten their legs, tilting over them with extended arms and lengthened spines. When the voice describes the suicide of the young wife, the dancers stop for a moment; each drops her torso and head to the side, one arm flopping downward while the other extends to suggest death by hanging.

Following this pause, the duet's movement becomes more panicked. The dancers twitch through hand gestures, jump suddenly, and catapult to the floor. The soloist, who up till now had seemed to be in a trancelike state, joins in with frantic gesticulations and short, skittish bursts of running. In her frenzy, she lets the bridal shawl drop. After the duo exits, the soloist halts and puts the veil on again. Her hands meet at her chest in a prayer position. Her elbows straighten as she raises her hands over her head, chanting "Agni Sati."[36] She varies the speed and emotion of the recitation, building it into a crescendo. Her hands wilt and fall. The rest of her body follows, and she collapses.

A video screen appears upstage, with a slow-motion shot of bangles falling to the floor.[37] The camera travels through a sparsely furnished bedroom, following which the video cuts to footage of a young girl. Meanwhile, three dancers materialize before the screen. Squatting, they reach up to it before turning to face the audience. They inch along the stage in this crouched position, hands combing the floor. One reaches over another and finds the bridal shawl. When she puts the garment down again, she looks underneath it and then stares at her hand. The other two dancers follow suit, gazing at their hands, nonplussed. The trio turns away from the veil and retreats back toward the screen.

The video images cease when one dancer rises and launches a sequence of powerful, articulate footwork. The other two dancers join her, and the trio performs grounded, staccato phrases. The ensemble breaks up into duets and solos, with one dancer leading and the other two framing her heavy, downward attacks with low extensions of legs and reaching arms. They strike the floor with swift, powerful impact, replacing the ornate, graceful arm positions of the classical forms with extended limbs that slice through the air and wrists that flex suddenly. The lone dancer picks up the veil and tosses it over her shoulder. She reaches her hand upward, with wrist and fingertips pointing back, still sinking into a turned-out, bent-leg position. She lowers her arm sharply and suddenly so that her raised palm seems to say "stop." She freezes in this pose. The duo splits and the dancers line up one behind another. One extends her arms to the side and takes a wide, rotated stance. The third dancer stands with arms upraised. The piece ends with the performers joined in this powerful stillness.

Unable to Remember Roop Kanwar points to the difficulty of representing the sati without turning her into an overdetermined, monolithic symbol of the abject "Third World Woman" (Spivak 1988: 296). It directs the audience's attention to the struggle to name oppressive practices without capitulating to neocolonial sensationalism. Chatterjea's piece, by commenting upon the impossibility of representing Roop Kanwar, unravels the conflation of subjectivity and representation with reform and revival. The choreography raises the vexed concerns of subjectivity construction that the consolidation of "respectable femininity" masks. The bhadramahila united reformist and revivalist discourses into a single model of circumscribed agency. The sati confounds this project. Both defenders of sati and feminists have claimed to represent the sati's will by pointing to voluntary decisions and to coercion or a lack of options, respectively (Rajan 1993: 18–19, 21). Reconstruction of the sati's subjectivity remains unachievable, however, precisely because the sati's death "creat[es] a condition of definitional unknowability" (Rajan 1993: 26). The sati thus splits the convergence of subjectivity and representation apart so that the very reconstruction of her will becomes both a point of contestation and an impossibility.

By replacing a resolution with a multiplicity of only partially answered women's questions, Chatterjea's piece eschews an ex-nomination of gender concerns that would universalize the choreographer's own subject position. It sheds light on the subject- as well as object-producing projects of revivalist pieces such as *Stree Shakti* as well as of reformist choreographies such as *Kanya* and *In Search of Devi*. By bringing the double bind of representation to the fore, *Unable to Remember Roop Kanwar* indicates the extent to which the new avenues for self-representation that have emerged in classical Indian dance in the twentieth century nonetheless continue to rest upon colonial gender discourses.

At the same time, Ananya Chatterjea offers an alternative to this need-to-represent/cannot-represent bind. She concludes the narrated section with a commemoration of resistance, ending the work with a visualization of oppositional force through the powerful footwork of Indian classical dance and through strong, direct arm gestures. In demonstrating struggle through the dynamics of classical phrases, Chatterjea's piece offers alternatives to customary representations of women as either self-sacrificing heroines or victims of an oppressive system. This portrayal of resistance opens up other options for contesting gender inequity. Struggle replaces both reform and celebration so that feminism does not need to recover autonomous subjects to find oppositional action. Resistance highlights the specific, the immediate, and the small-scale so that feminism can avoid universalizing narratives of either repression or valorization. Defiance, as a critical device, allows a dance practitioner to articulate broader political discourses in such a way that they unsettle the conventional subject-object model through which Indian women and Indian classical dance have been customarily represented.

Unable to Remember Roop Kanwar challenges gender oppression through struggle, not through resolution. Chatterjea takes a different approach from that offered by Visweswaran, who celebrates agency, or Madhuvanty, who urges reform and the remaking of marginal women. Like Sarabhai, Chatterjea rejects a victim-agent dichotomy. *Roop Kanwar*, however, addresses its international situation more directly than *In Search of Devi*.

By positioning sati alongside other, less spectacularized and exoticized forms of violence against women, Chatterjea's work foregrounds the oppressive practices of its North American audience as well as those located in Indian villages. The piece interrogates its own global situation and the transnational positioning of Indian classical dance forms. It suggests that Indian classical dance forms already inhabit a resolutely transnational sphere and suggests ways for these practices to grapple with the concerns of their immediate environment. Such work frames up the ability of classical dance not only to speak to political issues but also to address new local contexts.

4: The Production of Locality

Displacement, Urbanization, and the Colonial Local

Much as bharata natyam seems initially to be essentially feminine, it also gives the impression of retaining strong local ties. Replete with markers of tradition and continuity, it almost goes without saying that the dance form emerged from a particular place and maintains links to the same. If bharata natyam has roots that extend back centuries, then it seems to follow that these roots must tie it to a specific place.

Bharata natyam's relationship to its place of origin, however, is more complex than this first impression would suggest. Just as twentieth-century choreography established itself in relation to its past, its refiguration also depended on where it belonged in space and how it belonged through changing political circumstances. The shift of bharata natyam and Carnatic music in the nineteenth and twentieth centuries from the towns and villages of the Thanjavur region to the public concert halls of Madras developed out of economic, social, and political transformations. The dance form underwent several displacements before its appearance on the modern concert stage. These disruptions emerged out of shifts in local economic systems and ideology caused by imperialism. Although the production of belongings for bharata natyam articulated itself most obviously through large-scale political discourses such as nationalism and regionalism, these strategies also allowed dancers to contend with the urbanization of Indian arts and their global circulation.

This chapter investigates the localizing processes that established bharata natyam in Madras, on the one hand, and in international cities, on the other. As in the case of nationalism, regionalism, and gender identity, dancers deployed tactics that installed bharata natyam in its new home—the concert stage of Madras—in negotiation with the city's hybridity as a former colonial center. This process began with the shift of non-Brahman arts patronage to Madras in the early nineteenth century, accelerated with the establishment of sabhas in the late nineteenth century,[1] and consolidated itself further through Brahman patronage in the early twentieth century. The eradication of dance in temples driven by the anti-nautch movement confirmed the repositioning of bharata natyam by separating dance from ritual and court contexts (Srinivasan 1983, 1985).

From the 1920s to the 1940s, dancers contended with the displacement of bharata natyam from the villages and towns of southern India and participated in the urbanization of classical performance by affiliating the dance form with Madras. Practitioners and promoters made provision for concerts and training in Madras through the establishment of venues, concert series, and bharata natyam schools as well as through changes in choreography, instruction, and discourses on dance. These changes established Madras, not so much as a physical entity, than as a space, a place experienced through practice (Certeau 1988: 117). The refiguration of bharata natyam in the early twentieth century as a classical form in turn reinforced the establishment of Madras as an arts center.

Yet the relationship between bharata natyam and Madras did not only affiliate the dance form with the city; it also enabled bharata natyam to establish itself beyond this specific urban environment and to integrate itself into the cultural life of other metropolitan centers. The move from multiple sites of practice to a single one reversed itself in the late twentieth century. From the beginning of the postcolonial period, bharata natyam spread from Madras to other Indian cities, through pedagogical relationships and institutions as well as through the formation of state arts venues and organizations such as the National Centre for Performing Arts in Bombay (renamed Mumbai in 1995) and Sangeet Natak Akademi in Delhi. The globalization of Indian communities and the transnational networks that established modern dance and ballet as high art in Europe and North America further accelerated the circulation of bharata natyam choreography in the late twentieth century. Having previously negotiated hybridity, bharata natyam came to accommodate increasingly complex productions of identity in transnational, non-Indian cities.

Bharata natyam contains choreographic devices and accompanying discursive descriptions that align place, performance, and belonging. Eighteenth- and nineteenth-century songs invoked local affiliation through depictions of place, celebrations of specific cities and temples, and the valorization of gods and kings of particular areas, idioms that cultivated sentiments of belonging by associating the dance form with particular communities and environments. The choreographic legacy of bharata natyam also bears the traces of localizing when, for instance, styles are identified by the towns and villages that they come from (Thanjavur, Pandanallur, Vazhuvoor). Although images of place and space produced local identifications, even these relationships of choreography to context were not organic or unselfconscious because such references articulated themselves in relation to changing political circumstances.

Dancers, musicians, and scholars refer to the city of Thanjavur and its environs as the seventeenth-, eighteenth-, and nineteenth-century center of dance and music (Seetha 1981: 8) and, thus, as the ancestral home of bharata natyam and Carnatic music. However, migration and social upheaval facilitated the convergence of music and dance performance on Thanjavur. This first wave of the consolidation of the arts emerged out of intercultural exchange and of colonial modernity. The burgeoning of artistic production in the seventeenth to nineteenth century appeared under the rule of non-Tamil kings, first the Telugu Nayaka rulers (fourteenth to seventeenth century), followed by the Maratha regents (1674–1855).[2] Both eras saw an increased interest in and patronage of literature and performance, with creative practices forming a response to both upheaval and exchange (Peterson 2001). As the music historian Lakshmi Subramanian (2006) notes, the growth of a contemporary sensibility, inflected by colonial ideologies and by intranational cultural hybridity, sparked artistic production in eighteenth-century southern India. These intersections, Subramanian argues, resulted in the emergence of a modern classical tradition.

The transference of dance and music performance from Thanjavur to Madras, like their consolidation in Thanjavur, occurred through large-scale migrations, cross-cultural interactions, and alterations in ideology and economics through colonialism.[3] This transition did not hinge upon a single event but rather took place over several centuries. Indira Viswanathan Peterson argues that by 1800 Madras had emerged as a "new and different type of urban formation" because of its intersection with colonial economic institutions (2001: 2). Following Susan Neild Basu, Peterson maintains that the patronage of *Vellalas*—upper-caste non-Brahmans—drew performing artists to Madras. The Vellalas, wealthy landowners and agriculturalists, took up positions as *dubashes*, or middlemen—agents, brokers, managers, and bankers—to the British East India Company (Peterson 2001: 3). Prosperous Vellalas had already acted in rural areas as patrons of music, dance, and literary production, and they brought this function with them when they assumed new roles in the Madras economy (Peterson 2001: 23). Through this sponsorship, Madras emerged as an artistic center, a process that anticipated the recontextualization of classical performance in Madras by Brahman dancers, musicians, and promoters in the late nineteenth and early twentieth centuries.

Peterson reconstructs the burgeoning importance of Madras as an arts center through the depiction of performance and sponsorship in a nineteenth-century Sanskrit manuscript entitled *Sarvadevavilasa*. The narrative describes the growing importance of Madras's cultural life, identifying the social and political transitions that established the city as a center for dance, music, and literature in the eighteenth and nineteenth centuries. Raghavan discovered the text in 1939 while researching the history of Madras (Peterson 2001: 4). He produced a commentary on it in 1945, entitled "Some Musicians and Their Patrons about 1800 A.D. in Madras City," then edited and published the Sanskrit text in 1958. *Sarvadevavilasa* describes the city and its performances, celebrating the role of the dubashes in bringing together cultural practitioners from outside the city and in sponsoring their performances (Peterson 2001: 18). The tale portrays the cultural milieu of Madras through two Brahmans' search for patronage in the developing urban center. In the process, the two characters encounter performances at homes and in festivals, including those by the courtesan singers and dancers associated with Madras temples. The *Sarvadevavilasa* confirms that the importance of Madras as an artistic hub predated the anti-nautch movement and the classical dance and music revivals. Moreover, as Peterson argues, the text's attention to public performances prefigured the emergence of Madras's sabhas and consolidated an early urban modernity in the arts (2001: 25).[4]

Whereas colonialism enabled the development of patronage systems in Madras, it dismantled them in Thanjavur. The British East India Company eroded the power of the Thanjavur kings, finally eradicating it completely with British Empire's assumption of direct rule in 1858. As Krishnan (2004) and Meduri (1996) indicate, the colonial annexation of the Thanjavur region destroyed the patronage networks that supported dance by disempowering the rajas who sponsored court performance and funded the temples of their region. Matthew Allen maintains that direct colonial rule not only unraveled the patronage structures that provided backing for dance and music performances, but also eradicated an entire "context for interpretation" (1998: 36, 41). Both Krishnan and Meduri suggest that the British incursion into southern Indian prompted the standardization of dance performance by the Thanjavur Quartet in the early nineteenth century. Krishnan further argues that this interest in standardization, identified as a high point of dance history, constituted a response to the perceived demise of the devadasi dance tradition (Krishnan 2004). This destruction of Thanjavur's patronage structures in turn prompted performers to converge upon Madras (Allen 1998: 41).[5]

In the late nineteenth and early twentieth centuries, power and patronage changed hands, with Brahmans ascending to prominence through government civil service positions (Irschick 1986: 21; Peterson 2001: 26). These upper-caste communities pursued a Western education, attuned themselves to governmental politics, and remained keenly conscious of their subordinate status in the colonial hierarchy.[6] Therefore, as Indira Peterson (2001) and Lakshmi Subramanian (2006) indicate, the development of a new middle-class arts-consuming public, whose perspectives were informed by colonialism and nationalism, facilitated the shift of dance and music from Thanjavur to Madras. This community applied new meanings to cultural consumption and turned to the performing arts as a fundamental component of "cultural self-definition . . . and a cementing agent of a collective identity" (Subramanian 2004: 27), patronizing the sabha system and its network of private venues for music and dance performance as an extension of these interests. Conversely, as Allen argues, the consolidation of definitions of classicism and their articulation through music and dance performances at these sabhas enabled the development of a nationalist interpretation of the arts (1998:

25). The patronage and artistic activities of an educated, politically aware elite, as Allen (1998), Peterson (2001), and Subramanian (2004, 2006) indicate, contributed to the developed of a modern public sphere in Madras.

The anti-nautch movement consolidated rather than initiated the displacement and relocation of dancers and musicians. The anti-nautch campaign had sought to abolish dance in Hindu temples, as well as in other public and private venues, by eroding support for solo female dance in the multiplicity of towns and villages that had once fostered it. Although activists set out to address concerns of gender, domesticity, and religiosity, their campaign also furthered the urbanization of the arts in southern India, displacing sadir and severing a close relationship between choreography, context, and community. These agitations separated performance from ritual practice and removed sadir from the hands of devadasi practitioners, eradicating less the dances than the institutions that enabled their performance.[7] Devadasi dance in towns and villages had, by the 1930s, lost its social function and most of its structures of social and economic support. The abolition of temple dance and of the devadasi office accelerated the migration of performing artists from smaller towns to larger urban centers, especially to Madras (Gaston 1996: 57). Through the promotional activities of institutions such as the Music Academy and the instructional requirements of the new middle-class practitioners, the revival brought devadasi performers and, even more, their male counterparts to Madras, furthering a centralizing process that had begun a century before.

The revival encouraged dance practitioners to reestablish bharata natyam outside its places of origin and, through this reassociation, allowed them to differentiate their practice from that of devadasis. The dancers who reformulated sadir as bharata natyam, as Amrit Srinivasan (1983, 1985) suggests, predicated their refiguration upon this uprooting. Although this rupture validated upper-caste practitioners' forays into the dance field, it also required that performers find new affiliations for the dance practice and establish new kinds of relationships between choreography and context. Because of this interruption, then, the concert form required new, more explicit, and intentional localizing strategies.

At the same time that a number of economic, social, and political factors encouraged the convergence of classical dance and music on Madras, other circumstances encouraged the dance form outward, both intra- and transnationally. Sadir, and images of it, traveled domestically and globally before the bharata natyam revival, with, for instance, the Pondicherry devadasis dancing in London and Paris in 1838 and sadir dancers from Thanjavur joining the court of Maharaja Sarfoji Rao in the North Indian city of Baroda in the late nineteenth century (Kumar 1989: 21). The revival-era practitioners Ragini Devi and Balasaraswati performed at the 1934 All India Music Conference in Benares, an event that furthered the acknowledgment of bharata natyam in northern India (Gaston 1996: 83). Subsequently, Rukmini Devi and Balasaraswati, through performance tours, installed bharata natyam on a national level, which then sparked international interest in the dance form through instructional networks (Devi) and concerts and residencies (Balasaraswati).

Like his predecessor Uday Shankar, Ram Gopal turned the attention of mainstream dance viewers abroad to Indian forms. Gopal performed outside of India, in Southeast and East Asia, for the first time in 1936 (Khokar 2004: 37). While Rukmini Devi consolidated the respectability of bharata natyam by forming the Kalakshetra institution and Balasaraswati validated the dance form through performances in Madras and Benares, Gopal presented the classical form to an international viewership. He subsequently extended this project when he staged bharata natyam and other classical Indian dances not only at esteemed arts venues, but also at popular theaters, such as those of London's West End. As his precursor had, Gopal performed duets and group pieces and was recognized for his collaboration with a ballerina, Alicia Markova. Unlike Shankar, however, Gopal relied upon the classical form, making alterations to the length of pieces and the structure of an evening's concert rather than to movement vocabulary (Khokar 2004: 36, 37–38). Like Balasaraswati, Gopal enjoyed greater acclaim abroad than in India; he spent most of his life in London (38). Whereas Balasaraswati's emphasis on emotion and interior experience appealed to modernists both in India and abroad, Gopal continued the relationships between Indian dance and ballet that Shankar and Devi established.

The simultaneous dislocation of sadir from its earlier context and the intersection between bharata natyam and transnational discourses on dance encouraged dancers to look beyond the concerns of their immediate environment. The international circulation of dancers and choreography also challenged bharata natyam practitioners to relocalize the form in its new contexts. Contending on the one hand with the urbanization of arts and practitioners and on the other with a globalization of artistic concepts and performance careers, the revival's dancers deployed localizing strategies alongside historical, national, regional, and gendered ones. The bharata natyam revival hinged upon the ability of dancers and promoters to recontextualize a form that had been displaced and to find a place for it in an international dance milieu.

As I argued in chapter 2, divergent understandings of history allowed performers to align bharata natyam with specific communities. In this chapter, I suggest that these historical narratives, and their political resonances, also enabled dancers and promoters to respond to Madras's new position as an arts center and to the global circulation of the dance form. Practitioners thus introduced new kinds of social affiliation to choreographic and pedagogical practice.

Following Arjun Appadurai, I examine these affiliations as "structures of feeling" that contribute to immediate, as well as imagined, communities (1996: 181–82). Appadurai calls the sentiments that enable a sense of belonging to a social group "locality." Like Appadurai, I assume that identification does not arise au-

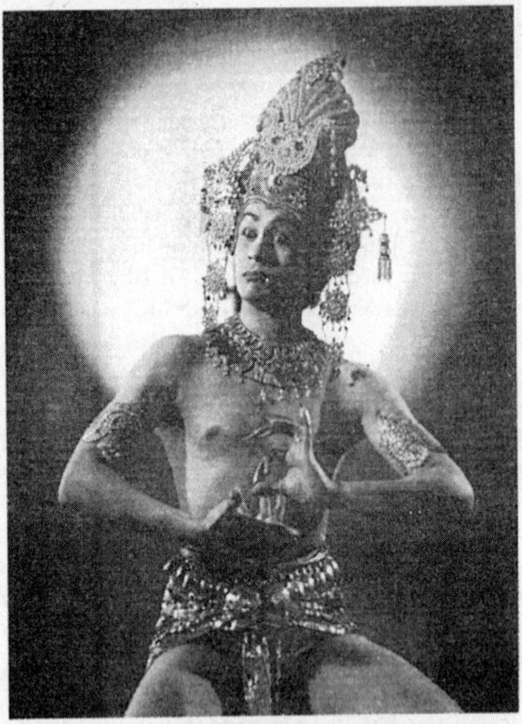

Figure 18: Ram Gopal. © V & A Images/Victoria and Albert Museum.

tomatically from participation in group life or from shared national, linguistic, or "ethnic" origins but must be cultivated actively, if not always explicitly. Divergent political contexts provoke varying constructions of the local that articulate themselves through contrasting strategies. Moreover, Appadurai's concept indicates that crises of cultural continuity not only bolster the need for allegiance, but also fundamentally alter the kinds of localizing strategies that a community requires: immediate, proximate groups construct their sense of the local differently from those that have witnessed ruptures in social affiliation through colonialism and diasporic migration. I therefore use the term locality to illustrate a self-aware production of urban identity in response to global political and economic forces. When I suggest that bharata natyam provides practitioners and viewers with devices for establishing locality, I refer specifically to the cultivation of community in choreography as it appears in response to the dance form's displacement from temple and court contexts and its reestablishment in the colonial center of Madras.

Bharata natyam rooted itself in Madras through the production of new local affiliations for the dance form. Localizing strategies appeared in choreography and in discourses around it; these changes served to affiliate bharata natyam with new communities of patrons and performers and with new kinds of viewership. At the same time, and especially in the late twentieth century, dancers and promoters used a range of strategies to contend with the international circulation of performers and dances. Thus, bharata natyam acquired the ability to both produce and transform local identities in a global context.

Choreographing Madras

Like the nation-state, former colonial centers grapple with a double identity. Produced by imperialist economic and governmental practices, they nonetheless incur responsibility for representing indigenous cultural identity. Colonial and early postcolonial cities such as Madras had, through their status as centers of colonial administration, the economic resources to support an arts milieu. In the absence of royal patronage, such commercial sites, with a solid middle class and a politically aware public, offered private support for the arts through sabhas. Its colonial legacy therefore enabled Madras to cultivate artistic forms that could be recrafted in the interest of a non-colonial past.

Both Kalakshetra and the Madras Music Academy, while refiguring bharata natyam in the interest of national pride, also affiliated the dance form with the city of Madras. Each institution came into being in large part because of their founders' political commitment to the ideal of the independent nation-state. Each also established bharata natyam in a relationship to a much more immediate community, in the urban center, through the abstract entities of the nation and the region. The two organizations encouraged a convergence upon Madras of practitioners from outside while also encouraging Madras residents to take up the form. Both organizations' approaches to pedagogy and performance, then, served to relocalize bharata natyam in Madras.

Some revival-era dancers, such as E. Krishna Iyer, traveled to smaller centers to study with Isai Vellala practitioners (Gaston 1996: 127–28). The trend of dancers pursuing training with Isai Vellala mentors in outlying areas continued through the twentieth century with, for example, Mrinalini Sarabhai, Shanta Rao, and Ram Gopal studying in Pandanallur village with Meenakshisundaram Pillai (Singer 1958: 370) and Vyjayantimala Bali and Hari Krishnan learning dance in Thanjavur under Kittappa Pillai. However, the revival also facilitated the more compelling reverse pattern of nattuvanars moving to major urban centers in order to teach larger numbers of students (Gaston 1996: 127–28). Rukmini Devi, for instance, invited Isai Vellala practitioners, most notably Meenakshisundaram Pillai, followed by his son Chokkalingam Pillai, to Kalakshetra to act as instructors.

This shift of nattuvanars to urban dance schools initiated one kind of convergence upon Madras, while Rukmini Devi's instructional and institutionalizing practices prompted another: the influx of dance students from a number of Indian cities and towns and, eventually, from all over the world to the Adayar district of Madras. Their presence and their performance practice contributed to the city's reputation as an authoritative center for bharata natyam. Some of Rukmini Devi's students set up schools elsewhere in India and internationally, but they remained affiliated with Kalakshetra, returning to Madras for further study, to perform, and to attend concerts. This allegiance supported Madras's position as the focal point for bharata natyam performance.

Rukmini Devi further augmented Madras's reputation as a cultural center through the institutionalization of dance training. When she legitimized dance for a national middle class by providing standardized instruction alongside formal academic education, Devi contributed to the centripetal pull of the Madras arts milieu by drawing outside students to the Adayar institution. Her aim of galvanizing and reinvigorating a diminished form likewise gave the Madras arts scene a further sense of purpose as over succeeding decades the city drew practitioners from other areas and therefore upheld a practice that was disappearing elsewhere.

The Kalakshetra syllabus system fostered an approach to pedagogy that could travel and yet continue to reference an original site of practice. Although Rukmini Devi initially expressed reluctance at teaching non-Hindus (Sarada 1996: 15), she came to welcome Indians of a range of religious and linguistic backgrounds and, subsequently, international students. Through foreign trainees and Indian disciples who relocate abroad, the Kalakshetra style circulates globally and roots itself internationally. Many Kalakshetra dancers remain associated with the school, teaching students internationally and sending them to the South Madras institute for further study, a process that has allowed Kalakshetra communities to spring up in cities throughout the world. This interest in continuity and standardization supports Kalakshetra as a style but also refers back to the institution in Chennai. The global dispersion of the Kalakshetra style thereby consolidates the city's importance as a center.

Like Rukmini Devi, the Music Academy's officers drew dance performance to Madras. However, just as the cultural and political investments of the Music Academy differed from that of Kalakshetra, so too did their localizing strategies. Whereas Kalakshetra embraced a pan-Indian cultural nationalism that rested on commonalities among a range of Indian forms, the Music Academy valorized regional practices as the foundation on which national pride rested. This attention to southern Indian affiliations alongside national ones found a parallel in the academy's promotion of performances from former regional centers in the new context of Madras. The Music Academy thus contributed to Madras's importance initially by sponsoring concerts by devadasi dancers. With the important exceptions of Mylapore Gowri Ammal and Balasaraswati, these devadasi performers came not from Madras but from South Indian towns such as Pandanallur, Kumbakonam, and Tirunelveli. When, in 1938, the Music Academy began sponsoring recitals by middle-class and upper-caste women and Madras-based dancers figured prominently in them, its series became more intracity focused. Whereas Kalakshetra established Madras initially as a site of training, the Music Academy presented the city as a focal point for dance performance.

The Music Academy venture that confirmed the status of Madras as an arts center was the creation of the annual music season. Beginning with the music conference and concert series that accompanied the Indian National Congress meeting in Madras in 1927, the annual festival expanded to become a citywide event, with a range of venues sponsoring programs on a daily basis. Aficionados founded other sabhas, which also came to offer performance series during the music season. The numbers of sabhas increased in the late twentieth century, and the music season spread across theaters and neighborhoods, including venues such as the centrally located Music Academy and Mylapore Fine Arts and extending to Krishna Gana Sabha in T. Nagar and Kalakshetra in the south of Chennai. The season is a focal point of the performance year for critics, performers, aficionados, scholars, and tourists. For those with a serious interest in—and the time for—the festival, the concerts become a feature of daily life: in order to present as many artists as possible, venues offer up to twelve hours of short concerts, each about one and a half hours, running from morning until evening. The visibility and prestige attached to these opportunities draws not only local but also national and international artists to the city, bolstering the status of Chennai while sparking or furthering artistic careers.

Critics and journalists, as well as performers and impresarios, contributed to the role of Madras as a cultural center. Matthew Allen (1998) maintains that the consolidation of connoisseurship in Madras, through the efforts of the Music Academy established Carnatic music as a modern classical tradition. Allen discusses several strategies, including the formation of an experts committee and the standardization of ragas, that the new community of connoisseurs deployed in order to establish the sabhas—and particularly the Music Academy—as authoritative sites of classical performance (1998: 42–43). Milton Singer (1958) indicates that the emergence of a specialist field of dance criticism facilitated the bharata natyam revival. Concert programming, changes to pedagogy, and the emergence of dance journalism facilitated the establishment of bharata natyam in its new context. Relying on Allen and Singer's arguments, I suggest that arts criticism not only fostered the development of a knowledgeable viewership, but also did so in relation to the status of Madras as a modern colonial center. The establishment of voluntary arts organizations together with the emergence of a separate field of dance and music criticism created a pool of erudite, articulate viewers reading and writing in English. This, together with the resources that Madras offered as an economic center, allowed the city to supplant the courts by cultivating a new kind of *rasika* (knowledgeable aficionado), one fluent in English and with access to print media, whose viewing experience is important to but also separate from daily life. Critical writing drew attention to both South Indian arts and the role of Madras in their development, both domestically and abroad. This phenomenon extends from South Indian arts publications such as *Sruti* and includes international periodicals. American performers and viewers learned of the reputation of Chennai through Sunil Kothari's coverage of the annual music season in such prominent dance publications as *Dance Magazine*. As a result, dancers and spectators, even those without a direct connection to bharata natyam, came to see Chennai as an arts center. This led to an international view of Chennai as an authoritative site of dance practice.

Balasaraswati, although closely associated with the Music Academy, highlighted the rupture as well as the consolidation that the revival and its resulting urbanization initiated. For Balasaraswati, the bharata natyam revival revealed the fracturing of an otherwise continuous tradition. As a result, she, even more than other practitioners, intimated that the dance belonged elsewhere than where it was currently performed. Nonetheless, her dance school at the Music Academy, her numerous performances in Madras, and her continued presence in that city helped to establish it as the dance form's new center. Furthermore, Balasaraswati's sense of loss in itself contributed to the role that Madras played as a focal point for bharata natyam. Because the idea of a disappearing dance practice in need of rescue gave Madras's patronage and performance activities their impetus, Balasaraswati, by signaling the decline of dance in its most "traditional" forms, bolstered the Madras arts community's raison d'être. Although Rukmini Devi's and Balasaraswati's perspectives on the dance form diverged, identifying the revival as either a reinvigoration or a loss, respectively, each of these points of view enabled the development of Madras as the new site of performance.

Despite her emphasis on regional traditions, Balasaraswati performed and taught internationally. As well as producing a core group of disciples in Madras, her instruction fostered a community of U.S.-based, primarily non-Indian, and almost exclusively non-Tamil bharata natyam dancers, a number of whom became long-term students and professional performers.[8] Balasaraswati offered her international students a paradigm of personal autonomy combined with a sense of history (Cowdery 1995: 56). Mediated through Balasaraswati's own view of the past, these women foregrounded the diminishing devadasi system, associating it with Balasaraswati's strength of personality and her status as a strong female role model "within a relatively clear set of gender expectations" (Renouf, quoted in Cowdery 1995: 54). These practitioners expressed an appreciation for Balasaraswati's paradoxical situation in which her unwavering allegiance to tradition reinforced her individuality and placed her outside of a rapidly changing bharata natyam milieu. Whereas Rukmini Devi established bharata natyam nationally and internationally through a pedagogical network, Balasaraswati created an international appreciation for bharata natyam through this sense of singularity.[9]

Balasaraswati provided her U.S. students with intensive training, but for many of them Chennai represented the ideal locus for dance study and, ultimately, performance. Although most of her foreign students visited Chennai but did not remain there, these North American dancers nonetheless contributed to Chennai's status as a dance center, traveling to the city for their own training and performance experience as well as sending their students there. This development of international interest in long-term bharata natyam tutelage bolstered Chennai's reputation as a center for and source of bharata natyam. Balasaraswati's instructional endeavors therefore established bharata natyam internationally by producing knowledgeable viewers, performers, and teachers based outside India. Her teaching helped consolidate bharata natyam's international status at the same time that this global interest supported Madras's reputation as a center for bharata natyam training and performance.

Madras's dancers reinforced the new site of practice not only through promotion and instruction, but also through composition. Rukmini Devi, for instance, created dance works that paralleled Madras's own hybridity, blending southern Indian practices with pan-Indian themes and infusing both with influences from Sanskrit and European theatrical traditions.[10] She did not have to negotiate a rupture in the dance practice's function because for her bharata natyam had existed for centuries in many different forms; the devadasi period represented only one aspect of that long history. Just as her broad sense of history enabled innovation by demonstrating the inevitability of change, it also allowed the past to feed into bharata natyam's appearance in Madras.

Devi's dance dramas accommodated regional, national, and international elements that reflected and supported Madras's status as a site where transregional and transnational influences intertwined. Her kuravanjis, as much as they provided a means of negotiating the imperatives of innovation and tradition, also offered a paradigm for intertwining elements that Indira Viswanathan Peterson labels "transregional and multilingual" (1998: 66). Peterson, in her investigation of the kuravanji genre, locates the dance drama's "heterogeneous origins" (43) in the polyglot, multicultural environment of the seventeenth- and eighteenth-century Tamil courts, in which Telugu and Marathi rulers established their own positions through the representation of folk traditions. In drawing together divergent group identities—folk and classical; Tamil, Telugu, and Marathi—these dance dramas authorized the court's position in relation to the diverse populations of Tamil Nadu (Peterson 1998: 48–49).

Although Rukmini Devi interpreted the relationship between the folk and the classical differently than her eighteenth-century counterparts did (Peterson 1998: 59), she retained the kuravanji's cross-regional qualities and its resulting cultural hybridity. The kuravanji of the twentieth century, like its earlier interpretations, offered its viewers, patrons, and performers a means of responding to a changing cultural context. As Peterson suggests, the twentieth century has seen a reclassicizing of the folk within the kuravanji genre (68), but these dance dramas nonetheless retained the ability to establish an urban center through the negotiation of Tamil and non-Tamil aesthetics. The eighteenth-century court performances operated as a paradigm for the modern kuravanji; Rukmini Devi's kuravanjis, in turn, articulated Madras's position as the site where cultures engaged with one another. The kuravanji's fusion of elements from a variety of Indian cultures spoke to Madras's status not only as a border town in which Tamil and Telugu cultures met but also as an arts center to which performers, students, and viewers traveled from other parts of India. In addition, when Devi supplemented her dance dramas with the compositional devices of Sanskrit drama and European stage techniques, she bolstered the position of Madras as a modern, cosmopolitan city. The inclusion of Sanskritic aesthetics contributed to the common national culture that Devi privileged, while the inclusion of European theatrical technologies and compositional strategies fostered a classical artistic culture that mirrored Madras's colonial past and thus its hybridity; similarly, the inclusion of European devices paralleled the engagement with colonial modernity that, as Lakshmi Subramanian (2006) argues, Carrnatic music incorporated in the eighteenth and nineteenth centuries. Such practices staged an identity for Madras as the point at which the multilingual regional, the national, and the global met.

For Balasaraswati and her supporters, by contrast, a continuous but threatened oral tradition led up to present-day bharata natyam, with nineteenth-century sadir constituting the high point of this practice. Although Balasaraswati regretted the loss of the Thanjavur legacy, she also established Madras through choreography that cultivated a sense of continuity. For example, V. Raghavan composed the lyrics and music for a dance piece, *Kalpakambal Sabdam*, which Balasaraswati performed and taught to her disciples, including Raghavan's daughters Nandini Ramani and Priyamvada Sankar. This sabdam praises the goddess Parvati in the peacock form that she takes at the Kalpaleshwarar temple of Madras's Mylapore district. The piece follows the musical and choreographic structure of a traditional sabdam, mobilizing the standard tropes of classical bharata natyam to praise a deity in a specific architectural and natural landscape. The choreography and lyrics describe the iconic forms of the goddess and the location of the temple, positioning this devotional recitation in relation to Mylapore rather than the religious and performance sites of the Thanjavur region more conventionally invoked in bharata natyam choreography.

Mylapore is a middle-class neighborhood with a large Brahman population that revolves, culturally and spatially, around its temple; the neighborhood began as a temple village (Singer 1958). Like the references to the great temples of the Thanjavur region in other, older items of repertoire, *Kalpakambal Sabdam*'s invocation of this area reinforces the devotional aspect of the choreography. The composition suggests historical continuity by using devices identical to those that were used to portray the Thanjavur area's temples in eighteenth- and nineteenth-century compositions. Like the dubashes, described in the *Sarvade-*

vavilasa, Raghavan and Balasaraswati, through *Kalpakambal Sabdam*, "dr[e]w upon their roots in older spatial and cultural locations, and on older traditions of worship [and] piety" (Peterson 2001: 21), molding "these traditional performances to new urban agendas and sensibilities" (24). This sabdam, therefore, intertwined a long-standing, continuous tradition with a new space and the experiences of new communities of spectatorship and performance.

Each of these participants in the bharata natyam revival contributed to the establishment of Madras as an arts center by mobilizing devices and images that linked bharata natyam's current position to its past. The status of Madras as a performance hub, in each interpretation, depended on its ability to accommodate multiple histories and influences. In several of these representations, Madras operated not only as a site of historical development, but also as a location where global forces grounded themselves. In the early twentieth century, Madras linked hybridity and history.

Performing the Translocal City

Although institutional and choreographic practices of the early twentieth century established Madras as a center where national, regional, and global concerns came together, the 1980s and 1990s carved out a different role for the city, renamed Chennai. In late twentieth century, Chennai provided bharata natyam with two functions. First, the city operated as the site of origin for an increasingly globalized dance form. The revival installed bharata natyam in Chennai successfully enough that, especially as figured from outside, bharata natyam belongs there. By the 1980s and 1990s, Chennai's reputation had solidified, and the city offered stability and constancy in the midst of accelerated transnational exchange. Chennai, by the late twentieth century, had provided the dance form with its source. Second, Chennai's ability to accommodate, through bharata natyam, translocal and transnational flows of dancers and choreography allowed bharata natyam to install itself in more globalized metropolitan centers.[11] The institutions and choreographies that developed Madras as a center for dance performance and training provided a paradigm for the installment of the dance form in other cities. The imperative for bharata natyam shifted from reconciling a singular, colonial hybridity into negotiating increasingly cosmopolitan social landscapes.

E. Krishna Iyer, V. Raghavan, Balasaraswati, and Rukmini Devi, among others, created and supported institutions dedicated to the propagation of classical arts that established Madras as an authoritative center for bharata natyam. The number of such venues and schools proliferated in the late twentieth century, and now a network of instructional institutions characterizes Chennai. The ubiquity of training institutions and theatres dedicated to the propagation of classical arts such as bharata natyam encouraged the participation of Chennai residents in the dance form, prompted a convergence of outside dancers upon the city, and guaranteed a continuous presence of dance and performers there. The presence of luminary teachers likewise assured that many dancers who became professionals remained in Madras even if they did not originally hail from there.

Although other cities acquired renown for bharata natyam pedagogy and performance, Chennai retained its primacy. Despite this authoritative role, however, Chennai's position as a late-twentieth-century arts center relied upon translocal, and often cross-national, pedagogical relationships. Bharata natyam, from the revival period onward, has stimulated the interest of dance practitioners based abroad. Dancers from both within and outside diasporic South Asian communities have contributed to the dance form's international reputation. The foreign dancers who traveled to Chennai for dance study included not only those trained through the dance networks established by Balasaraswati and Rukmini Devi, but also performers such as Ragini Devi, Nala Nalajan, and Bruce Murray Turner. Turner's practice of Indian dance led him to relocate to Delhi to facilitate his opportunities for performing in India. Likewise, dancers from diasporic Indian communities travel to Chennai for further tutelage and to perform. This global dispersion of the form established bharata natyam in new centers at the same time that it turned international attention toward Chennai.

Although the gurusishya system of continued study with one mentor remained an ideal, instructional relationships established in Chennai reach across geographical boundaries. Student dancers, especially those based abroad, supplement their training by studying with several mentors in the same instructional lineage but in different locations. Because Chennai plays such an important role in the bharata natyam milieu, dancers often desire immersion in that city's life as much as they seek intensive dance training. Physical distance creates a situation in which the imperatives of uninterrupted tutelage with one mentor and absorption into the Chennai milieu vie with one another.

Moreover, this interest in cultural reproduction creates a pool of young dancers who express their dedication to dance and their affiliation with their communities less often through an extended performance career and more frequently through arangetrams. Historically, the arangetram inaugurated a dancer's professional life, marking a young devadasi's entrance into ritual service and performance (Gaston 1996: 229). The late-twentieth-century arangetram, by contrast, signified amateur accomplishment, often terminating rather than launching a dancer's career, with student and teachers characterizing the arangetram as a "graduation" from a period of dance tutelage. The arangetram, which is frequently better attended than other bharata natyam concerts, presents the dancer to an audience consisting of friends, family, neighbors, and business associates of her parents rather than to a general dance community, or even an Indian classical dance subset of that sphere. Internationally, especially in the United States, the arangetram has also become a rite of passage that marks the entry of an adolescent girl into an Indian community (Greenstein and Bharadvaj 1998), substantiating her Indianness before her geographically proximate group of friends and relatives.[12] The diasporic arangetram brings together an immediate South Asian community, symbolizes cultural continuity in the face of physical distance, and confirms a young woman's belonging to a community that shares an allegiance to the culture of a homeland.

As much as late-twentieth-century arangetrams set bharata natyam up in international cities and towns, they still referenced Chennai as bharata natyam's origin point. Under the rubric of transnational pedagogical networks, young dancers traveled to Chennai for long-term, intensive bharata natyam study that led to arangetrams or other performances within the city. Although young dance pupils may have treated these periods of tutelage as an immersion in the rigors of dance training, their parents often characterized such terms of sustained practice as exposure to traditional Indian culture. Even when dancers could not hold their debuts in Chennai, some advertised the event in Chennai's renowned arts journals such as *Sruti*. These dancers and their supporters see Chennai as a site not only for dance, but also for a more authentic cultural life than that provided by their international position. This assumption fixes Chennai as a site of unchanging tradition. At the same time, this international imagining of a dance homeland also prompts the global circulation of dancers.[13] An interest in Chennai encourages travel to that city, which in turn contributes to the transformation of the dance milieu and of choreographic practice.

This focus on bharata natyam, on both local and international levels, encouraged late-twentieth-century dancers to seek out performances as well as training in Chennai. These concerts offered dancers a chance to perform before aficionados and to promote their work to a large and active dance community. Because a major effect of the move of dance and music practice to Madras and the establishment of venues was the (re-)cultivation of connoisseurship in the new urban center (Allen 1998; Subramanian 2006), dancing in Chennai presents dancers with knowledgeable viewers. This is especially important for international artists. Many diasporic and non-Indian bharata natyam dancers based abroad perform in mainstream dance milieus whose audiences have a limited understanding of classical South Asian forms, their music, their accompanying poetic texts, and their literary and religious heritage. Dancers who perform in such contexts spend much of their career explaining the dance form as well as dancing.[14] Concerts in Chennai bolster the credibility of dancers as performers, teachers, and choreographers within their local communities. Late-twentieth-century dancers, including internationally based ones, pursued performance opportunities, particularly during the music season, since these concerts tend to be among the best attended, most renowned, and the most publicized dance events. Reviews of these concerts also have a wider circulation than those of nonfestival events.

However, the same institutional operations that established Chennai as a center for bharata natyam have also urged dancers outward, away from that city, to look for further performance prospects. On the one hand, dancers gain cultural capital by performing in Chennai. Once Chennai achieved an authoritative status, dancers, no matter where they are based, began to seek out concerts in that city. On the other hand, performers rarely receive from these appearances the economic reimbursement needed to sustain a performing career.[15]

Since the late twentieth century, Chennai has housed a surplus of proficient dancers; these numbers swell during key points in the performance calendar such as the annual festival season. The majority of these dancers aim for a solo career, which, in turn, augments the effects of this surfeit. Moreover, because this surplus has inundated viewers with bharata natyam productions, venues can rarely promise attendance at dance events unless they offer free or inexpensive tickets. As a result, they often provide honoraria insufficient to cover the costs of planning a concert such that, for all except the most renowned dancers, reimbursement appears token. In setting up a concert, a bharata natyam dancer incurs costs that extend beyond the use of her own time. These expenses range from the purchase of a costume to the payment of the musical ensemble, the latter of which usually consists of four or five performers. The production of a group piece exacerbates these difficulties, because of the need to pay a cast of dancers, lighting designers, and musicians for rehearsals and performances. This situation, in which dancers require Chennai concerts but do not find financial reward in them, contributes to further peregrinations on the part of dancers and dances.

Nonetheless, competition has remained intense for these much-needed opportunities. Dancers, especially young and inexperienced ones, accept low-paying performance slots or those offering no reimbursement at all. In more extreme cases, dancers or the parents of young dancers agree to make a donation to the venue in exchange for a performance.[16] Sabhas, as privately funded institutions, depend on donations, memberships, and corporate sponsorship; thus, it follows that they tend to promote dancers who attract further support.

Dancers have adopted a number of strategies in order to contend with these pressures. Chennai performers who accept insufficient funding for their performances turn elsewhere for economic support, often choosing instruction as the means to self-sufficiency. Performers also supplement intracity concerts with outside ones, frequently turning to the better-paying international venues to support their career in Chennai because of the discrepancy between their payment policies and those of their Chennai counterparts.[17] Likewise, the Chennai-based dancers who procure such performance prospects benefit from currency imbalances, because they receive payment on U.S., European, or East Asian terms. If they plan their tours skillfully, they return to Chennai with a financial surplus that, when transferred into local currency, could fund other performances and ensemble productions.

Similarly, nonresident Indians and foreign performers, especially those from

Europe, North America, and East Asia, can use their access to hard currency to gain performance opportunities in Chennai. Internationally based dancers find the risk of economic loss worth taking because of the disparity between the wages they receive internationally and the cost of a Chennai concert. Dancers who remain in Chennai incur a dual economic burden because of these transactions. Performers from abroad who pay venues increase the stakes for local dancers whose resources, although often sufficient by local standards, do not benefit from augmentation by global currency imbalances. At the same time, venue directors, because of the international circulation of dancers and their works, may assume that local performers acquire funds from international tours. Such material concerns combine with the cultural capital that Chennai offers so the global patterns of import and export of dance through this city accelerate. Venue policies send dancers out in search of international support, while the cultural value of a Chennai performance assures that they continue to return. The global financial imbalances that inform bharata natyam's circulation have altered Chennai's social and choreographic landscape while reproducing it as a center.[18]

If global economic inequities are reinstalling Chennai as a center, dance festivals at temples seem to destabilize the urbanization process that the revival initiated.[19] In the 1980s and 1990s, impresarios began to sponsor dance performances in temples, describing them as a reinstallation of the religious function of the dance. Nagaswamy, the promoter of the annual Nataraja festival in Chidambaram, represented the event as a "return" to the temple performance context (Gaston 1996: 39). However, this festival does not involve ritual practice. It takes place outdoors, with dancers performing to an audience, in the public enclosure of a temple complex, instead of before the deity as part of religious worship. The occasion remains largely separate from both the temple's ritual practice and its community. Rather than drawing primarily upon a pool of local dancers, the Nataraja festival recruits performers largely from outside, and especially from Chennai.[20]

Although such festivals bring nonlocal dancers, critics, spectators, and some national and international tourists to towns like Chidambaram, outside dancers and aficionados do not integrate themselves into the fabric of the life of temple towns. Instead of bolstering bharata natyam's day-to-day existence in Chidambaram, then, the festival serves primarily to augment bharata natyam's role as a concert art in major cities such as Chennai while emphasizing its religious roots. Nagaswamy maintains that he promotes the festival for devotional and not touristic consumption;[21] however, the showcase presents such religiously oriented dances as part of a special occasion for dancers and viewers from Chennai, as well as from other Indian and international cities, rather than as part of the quotidian existence of the temple town.

Temple festivals draw urban dancers away from cities temporarily but ultimately bring them back to the civic center with a renewed sense of purpose. By highlighting bharata natyam's religious origins and therefore foregrounding a specific, validating aspect of its history, these events support the city's relatively new role as a dance center. At the same time, such occasions operate as a showcase for dancers and open the way to future performance opportunities back in the city, reinforcing the vitality of the arts center itself. Although performances take place at the temple, the role of Chidambaram remains largely symbolic. None of the older regional centers has the concentration of dance teachers or the economic resources to provide training on a large-scale level, and, thus, none rival Chennai as a site of artistic practice. Like the representation of Thanjavur in music discourses (Terada 2000), the Chidambaram festival references a "golden age" that validates present-day praxis rather than reestablishing dance in a nonurban site. Temple festivals position bharata natyam primarily as a concert, not ritual, art and thereby point to the need for knowledge and training that an arts center such as Chennai provides.

Although promotional activities distinguish dancers from one another on economic and geographical levels, with contrasts between international and domestic and between urban and rural coming to the fore, choreography offers opportunities for reconciliation between different groups. Dancers emphasize Chennai's transregional, polyglot, and multireligious qualities as the city's most apparent kinds of interculturality. The issues at stake in these works pertain less to class than to sociocultural difference, with dancers presenting work that foregrounds harmonious relationships between disparate groups. In the 1980s and 1990s, Chennai-based practitioners created works that encompassed multiple belongings through these kinds of affiliations.

In the 1980s, a collaborative performance genre known as the *jugalbandhi* rose to prominence. This format draws together two or more forms that stage themselves as distinct.[22] Basing the choreography on the structure of a classical repertory item, dancers of different forms combine analogous pieces into one work, juxtaposing rhythmical phrases from each dance style. Some of these pieces feature a duet at the end where the collaborators take the same rhythmic phrase, translate it into each dance vocabulary, and perform simultaneously but not in unison.

The jugalbandhi highlights regional difference in its fusion of forms. In this sense, it departs from Rukmini Devi's dance dramas, in which the features of bharata natyam and kathakali, although separate stylistically, contributed to an overall choreographic style. In Devi's work, kathakali and bharata natyam distinguished themselves primarily through a gendered division of choreographic labor: men used more of kathakali's wide stances and rocking torsos, while women retained bharata natyam's triangular leg positions. Performers of either sex employed kathakali's clear articulation of facial muscles in abhinaya. The two genres contributed to a unified, dramatic whole. In the jugalbandhi, by contrast, dancers compare and contrast two forms through their repeated juxtaposition. This format embodies a different vision of the intercultural city than that suggested by Rukmini Devi: in place of commonality, the jugalbandhi introduces parity in divergence. Although usually interpreted as a celebration of regional harmony and of unity-in-diversity nationalism, these pieces also establish the city as the site where divergent regional practices come together.[23] Through the jugalbandhi, the city emerges as the place where a nation-of-nations patriotism is practiced. The jugalbandhi forms part of a larger pattern: the production of local identities in choreography through the more abstract entities of the nation and the region.

A weeklong event entitled *Bharatam Samanvayam*, held in Chennai in September 1999, also fostered the idea of equality through difference. The promoters created the program in the interest of cultivating "religious concord and harmony" (program notes 1999) and foregrounding the message of tolerance espoused by all religions. Natyarangam, the sponsoring organization, commissioned dancers to perform pieces that celebrated the religions of India: Hinduism, Islam, Christianity, Buddhism, Sikhism, and Jainism. The majority of the presentations portrayed religious themes within such conventional genres as varnams and padams. In preparing for the event, the organizers paired dancers with scholars who located Tamil treatises on the particular faith. The dancers or their teachers then interpreted the themes of the text in choreography.

Bharatam Samanvayam, propagated as a defense of religion in response to political criticism, presented Chennai as a harmonious metropolis tolerant of difference. Although the series used solely Tamil-language texts and the bharata natyam movement vocabulary as its basis, it nonetheless projected a vision of urban interculturalism, articulated through religion rather than linguistic or regional identity. In drawing together the nation's faiths through bharata natyam's movement vocabulary and repertoire, the series suggests that the dance form's home city accommodates diversity, at least within the sphere of religion. This approach describes Tamil Nadu, and specifically Chennai, as "orthodox"—orthodoxy is here defined as adherence to religion—but inverts the customary valuation so that the traditionalism of this southern city correlates not to communalism but to an acceptance of difference. It establishes Chennai as a site where divergent elements and forces become localized and reconciled through dance.

Chennai's ability to negotiate translocal and transnational traffic through bharata natyam set the stage for the dance form's emergence in other international cities. There dancers have broadened choreographic dialogue to include other, non-Indian dance forms. Using dance forms such as flamenco and ballet, choreographers have juxtaposed stylistic elements of different practices and thus positioned bharata natyam in other intercultural environments that incorporate divergent ethnic, linguistic, and religious groups side by side. These choreographies establish the transnational city as the site where global pathways become localized.[24] Such works address the concerns of the metropoles of the former colonial powers and of North America, which consist of individuals who experience different kinds of rootedness at once (Bakht 1997: 8). Taking a cue from Chennai's translocal qualities, dancers integrate their practice into these multicultural cities.

In the process of staging new belongings, choreographers also challenge the marginalization of Indian classical dance. The San Francisco Bay Area choreographer Mythili Kumar receives local and national funding to show her work in prominent dance venues as well as through events sponsored by South Asian community organizations. Other choreographers, such as the Toronto choreographer Suddha Thakkar Khandwani, directly challenge mainstream biases against work that uses Indian classical dance forms. Khandwani created the Kalanidhi festival, dedicated to both classical and contemporary Indian dance, in order to rectify this situation, countering perceptions of stasis by illustrating the diversity and vibrancy of choreographic projects included in the category of Indian dance (personal correspondence 1999). Also in Toronto, the choreographers Lata Pada, Menaka Thakkar, and Hari Krishnan have brought their work to the Canadian contemporary dance field, using a range of choreographic strategies to align bharata natyam with other aesthetic systems and to render it comprehensible to a range of audiences. In London, dancers incorporated choreography based on Indian classical forms into performances at such prominent series as Dance Umbrella and Spring Loaded. In all these instances, dancers have used specific strategies that allow them to connect bharata natyam with a new center for training and performance.

The Toronto choreographer Lata Pada's *Cosmos* (1999) participates in a Canadian version of multiculturalism by drawing together, but not fusing, two different philosophical systems. As its name implies, *Cosmos* concerns itself with theories of universal creation. The piece opens on a semi-darkened, empty stage. A narrator, invisible but audible over the sound system, recites in English a passage from the Creation Hymn of the *Rig Veda* that reflects on the paradox of universal creation: "In the beginning there was nothing and there was not nothing." The unoccupied stage space reinforces the mysteriousness of the quote.

An ensemble of dancers bursts forth from the wings, perforating the charged vacuum with their dynamic, rhythmic phrases. The dancers careen through the space, winding their way into an increasingly tight spiral. They pause for a moment, tense in their stillness, then launch into a phrase of staccato footwork. As their percussive phrase impels them across the stage, the center appears to eject them outward. Their trajectories, linear at first, curve and intersect, becoming increasingly chaotic. The ensemble fractures into a collection of individual dancers, each of whom traces her own pathway after a "big bang" of explosive footwork. The dancers condense their traveling movements into parallel orbits, routes widening and flattening elliptically so that they cross one another without pushing each other off course. The dancers' trajectories begin to waver as though in

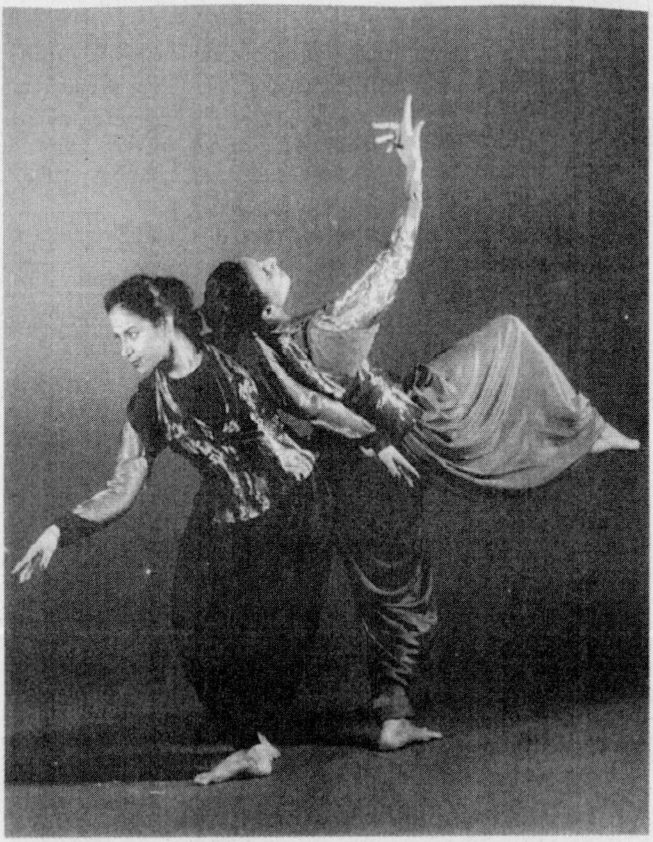

Figure 19: Lakshmi Venkataraman and Anandhi Narayanan in Lata Pada's *Cosmos*. Photograph by Cylla von Tiedemann.

response to some invisible force. The performers succumb to the pull of a black hole, resuming a pulsating phrase that indicates their increasing momentum as they catapult toward center stage.

Whereas earlier sections follow transitions from order to chaos and back again, the closing phrases evince the harmony of the solar system. The dancers develop cooperative relationships with one another, interweaving without colliding. They break off into duets. Back to back, they exchange weight, arms and hands arching into classical bharata natyam mudras as bodies remain taut and straight even in tilted positions. The stylized gestures and the dancers' stability reinforce the image of balance in the relationships between the relatively proximate planets.

Lata Pada's choreography depicts the creation of the universe by illustrating the churning of nebulous, primordial energy, its explosion into defined pieces of matter, and its compression into the specific orbits of heavenly bodies, blending the theories of creation put forth by European scientific traditions and by Vedic philosophy. *Cosmos* explains the two epistemological systems through one another, treating them as equivalent. By placing the Vedic hymn at the beginning of a depiction of the big bang, the work highlights the contradiction at the center of both the Vedic and scientific explanations of creation: each hypothesis suggests that matter arose from an undefined primeval force. Although Pada offers an English translation of the hymn, she nonetheless employs the South Asian text to demonstrate the paradox imbedded in the big-bang theory rather than using the cosmological hypothesis to argue for the rationality of the philosophical tract.

In addressing, through choreography, two different thought systems and treating them as equal but distinct, *Cosmos* inverts an Orientalist frame, interpreting the European epistemology through the Vedic philosophical one rather than vice versa. By integrating these two points of view, Pada not only indicates their conceptual similarities but also gestures to the global histories of both bharata natyam and Indian classical philosophy. In addition, by aligning but not blending distinct thought systems, so that they remain culturally identifiable, the piece positions bharata natyam in the hybrid landscape of the contemporary Canadian city. Canadian immigration and educational policies, in contrast to the U.S. melting-pot ideal, seek to preserve and harmonize cultural difference among various communities.[25] *Cosmos* therefore recalls the global pathways that constitute its local positioning, situating bharata natyam as an integral part of the urban environment. It contributes to a political climate that supports disparate elements engaging with one another but does not necessarily require that they merge.

Triple Hymn (2000), by Angika, a British dance company consisting of the dancer-choreographers Mayuri Boonham and Subathra Subramaniam, interweaves bharata natyam and Carnatic music with European classical music, integrating melodic, choreographic, and rhythmic components. To the sounds of a European operatic score, based on the words of the Sanskrit *Gayatri Mantra*, followed by a recitation of various names of Hindu goddesses, the two dancers render lyrical gestures from the bharata natyam movement vocabulary. During the *Gayatri Mantra* section, they perform symbolic mudras suggesting worship, prayer, and other ritual actions. They subsequently depict the various forms of the goddess through characteristic iconographic poses. They follow this with nonrepresentational phrases that extend the bharata natyam vocabulary through leg extensions, elevations, and arches of the torso.

The dancers highlight the religious aspect of bharata natyam but they do not restrict sacrality to the Indian form. Rather, the intersection of opera and religion evokes the transcendent qualities of both the European and the Indian practices. *Triple Hymn* places two signifiers of classicism—bharata natyam and European classical music—alongside each other. Boonham and Subramaniam link two traditions instead of interpreting one through the other, making explicit the cross-cultural exchange that fostered the project. The piece charts pathways of exchange moving in and through Britain but also opening out to both continental Europe and Asia. *Triple Hymn* speaks directly to the dynamic, cosmopolitan London environment in which it was performed.

Mythili Kumar's *In the Spirit* (1993) also draws two forms together without fusing them. *In the Spirit* has bharata natyam dancers performing staccato phrases of the classical dance form to the powerful accompaniment of San Jose Taiko, a Japanese drumming ensemble. Performed by Kumar's Abhinaya Dance Company, this piece aligns but does not blend two identifiably Asian forms. Although primarily an abstract, rhythmically based composition without overt dramatic context, the title invokes transcendence, suggesting a similarity between these forms in their relationship to spirituality. Both the presentation of the piece and its choreographic conjoining of rhythmic phrases highlight pan-Asian commonalities.[26]

The work's performance in San Jose, California, is not incidental. *In the Spirit* grounds a pan-Asian affiliation in a diverse local community, positioning bharata natyam as an integral part of a California social landscape that looks westward to Asia. It stages an Asian–Pacific Rim identity within its immediate social environment, highlighting an Asian presence in the San Jose area and Silicon Valley more generally. The piece speaks to long-standing economic and cultural links between California and Asia (including South Asia) as well as to growing economic connections between South and East Asia that connect India to the Pacific Rim. Kumar's piece also counters a tendency in the United States to overlook South Asians as part of the social identity category of "Asian" or "Asian American."[27] In abstract, nonnarrative form, it localizes the immigration patterns of middle-class professionals from Asia, foregrounding Asian spirituality for the San Francisco Bay Area's diasporic communities.

Each of these projects treats bharata natyam as an entity capable of responding to the hybridity of its immediate urban environment. Through bharata natyam, dancers establish social affiliations in the transnational city. Such work demonstrates the dance form's ability to underwrite the global positioning of its practitioners. The city emerges as a site for intercultural exchange, and bharata natyam enables these transactions. Through these investigations, bharata natyam provides a platform for dancers to represent their own transnational positions as they inform specific, local contexts.

Roger Sinha's Choreography of Unlocality

Rather than celebrate a diasporic identity as one of simultaneous belongings, the Canadian choreographer Roger Sinha's *Pehla Safar* (1994) depicts the migratory position as one of multiple exclusions. This piece, one of Sinha's early works, invokes "unlocality": Sinha makes explicit the dilemmas provoked by immigra-

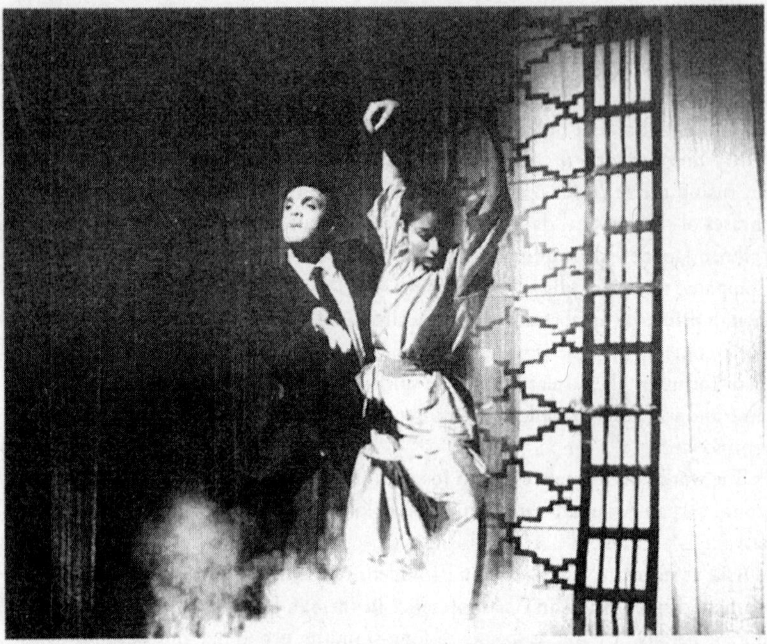

Figure 20: Roger Sinha and Natasha Bakht in *Pehla Safar*. Photograph by Stephen Hues.

tion and transnationalism and contests the vision of harmonious integration that Lata Pada, Angika, and Mythili Kumar put forth.[28] *Pehla Safar* (*First Journey*) opens with Sinha wearing a Western dress suit and carrying a suitcase, about to embark on an excursion. His travels lead him to a bharata natyam dancer, played by Natasha Bakht, who appears, literally, on a pedestal. He confronts his own Orientalist imaginings when the same dancer descends from the platform wearing a suit identical to Sinha's own. Nonetheless, Sinha pursues this elusive Indianness, trying imperfectly to imitate her movements as she switches between classical and hybrid movements and between European and Indian garb.

Sinha's pursuit of Indianness via bharata natyam does not result in the dance form and what it represents joining his world. Rather, he must go to it, and even then it eludes him. Bharata natyam here can only signify India, and an inaccurately imagined one at that. When Bakht demonstrates hybridity, for instance, she does so by moving out of the classical movement vocabulary entirely. *Pehla Safar* places bharata natyam in a global context but refuses any kind of relocalization. Although Sinha's piece deals largely with his own "unbelonging" (Roy 1997a), it also interrogates bharata natyam's ability to affiliate its practitioner with a non-Indian environment.

Pehla Safar diverges from the other works discussed here. It rejects bharata natyam's numerous rearticulations of the local and highlights the displacement of both form and practitioners. In treating bharata natyam as emblematic of Indianness, the choreography references the association of the dance form with intentional cultural reproduction on the part of nonresident Indian communities but treats this as a project that has failed. Sinha's approach contrasts with that of Lata Pada, Angika, and Mythili Kumar in that, for him, bharata natyam does not relocalize itself by blending with other forms, practices, or epistemologies and crafting a new multiculturalism. Rather, the dance form, for both the choreographer and, the work implies, his audience, remains in an exoticized position. Bharata natyam operates not as a device for self-representation, but as an icon that signifies an unattainable homeland.

This work concerns itself primarily with the choreographer's position as an Indian Canadian and his inability to belong either to a predominately Euro-Canadian community or to a resident South Asian one. His emphasis on bharata natyam's marginalization in a global dance milieu also points to the ruptures in the dance form's localizing strategies, shedding light on the rifts in other late-twentieth-century choreographers' cultivation of locality. On the one hand, this attention to the gaps in representation reminds Sinha's viewers that bharata natyam remains subject to colonial and neocolonial representations. On the other hand, the very deployment of this critique through choreography also points to the progressive and articulate potential of performance. Sinha's piece may reject relocalizing, but it continues to offer its choreographer and dancers an informed subject position from which to level a critique of dance and spectatorship in a transnational context. Bharata natyam, then, operates not a static tradition but as a dynamic force that challenges the assumptions of its practitioners and viewers.

Afterword: Toward a New Transnationalism?

This book arose out of my unease with conventional representations of bharata natyam as traditional and therefore fixed and unchanged. The divergence I witnessed within the form queried claims of seamless continuity and conformity. It also raised questions about the future of the dance form. Underlying this investigation into issues of continuity and transformation and their social, political, and economic implications are questions about what would come next, such as whether these competing visions needed to reconcile themselves or whether their tension was a productive one that would contribute to an increasingly vibrant field. In looking to that future, I raise two concerns that I hope will send this argument out in new directions. First, I return to the relationship between scholarship and choreography, which, in the field of bharata natyam, is a complex and mutually constituting one. Second, I want to consider what role bharata natyam's history will play in new articulations of the form.

The preceding chapters illustrate the social, cultural, political, and aesthetic contests that crafted bharata natyam's emergence as an urban concert practice. The debates that took place in broader social and political arenas affected decisions made within the choreographic sphere. Twentieth-century bharata natyam engaged with nationalist, regional, and Orientalist discourse, crosscut by concerns of a global dance modernism, debates over the status of women, and the urbanization of Indian arts. I have also suggested that late-twentieth-century choreographers negotiated between past and present, between nationality and transnationalism, and between local and regional identities. In the process, bharata natyam has become a dynamic, global practice characterized by local variation. The dance form has transformed and diverged during the last century, with changes escalating in the 1980s and 1990s.

As dancers, viewers, and writers, we are still in the process of developing a frame of reference that can keep pace with these varied interpretations of the dance form. In looking at bharata natyam's transformations over the last century, scholars and critics have tended to treat the burdens of history and politics as restrictive. There are good reasons for this: unpacking political discourse involves questioning ideological underpinnings and pointing out how dominant perspectives continue to reiterate themselves. However, the different directions in which bharata natyam has moved indicate the extent to which individuals claim ideologies in the interest of establishing their own subject positions and of creating meaning specific to their own local context. Although these subject positions remain vexed, they also reveal the political and aesthetic thoughtfulness that accompanies such self-fashioning.

In using this formerly marginal, nationally marked form to claim a position of representation, dancers disrupt the very hegemonic forces that act upon it. As problematical as these claims to subjectivity may be, they nonetheless allow performers to produce a different understanding of the dance form than its conventional interpretations initially yield. In the act of conceptualizing a choreographic statement, dancers take hold of an agency that, although troubled by broader political claims, nonetheless reveals patterns of resistance.

As they contended with concerns of nationhood and regional identity and with claims to tradition and to innovation, bharata natyam practitioners developed platforms for articulating their own views on the social and political concerns of specific, local, historical contexts. Dancers encountered a number of double binds: modernity and tradition, nationalism and universalism, cultural reproduction and invention. However, through this dance form, they grappled with these issues rather than simply reiterating them. This argument raises further questions about the creative and political potential of this form. If bharata natyam can establish and contend with concerns of the nation and the region, if it can express locality in an increasingly globalized world, and if it can negotiate gendered subjectivity, what other kinds of tasks can it undertake? As bharata natyam moves into its twenty-first-century articulations, its divergent social, political, and artistic meanings will require the development of new theoretical frames if viewership and scholarship are to keep pace.

The form may be entering another phase in which dancers once again reflect critically on its history. If the bharata natyam revival continued to inflect the practices of late-twentieth-century dancers, and if the practitioners of the revival deployed varied strategies, present-day dancers can look to the past in order to consider how these tactics could be reworked today, in response to a new set of social and political concerns. I want to suggest that the revival be reconsidered, neither to disparage or celebrate it, but to investigate it through a process that Mark Franko (1989) has identified as extracting the theoretical principles of a period in order to experiment with them.

Choreographers and scholars have already begun this process by rethinking the approach taken by Rukmini Devi. Research by Avanthi Meduri (2005b) suggests that Devi's approach be understood less as one of reconstruction and more as a modernist project. Similarly, Vena Ramphal argues that "while bharata natyam is so fond of Devi's rebellion it would do well to take more direct inspiration from it" (2003: 33). Shobana Jeyasingh maintains that Rukmini Devi's inquiries

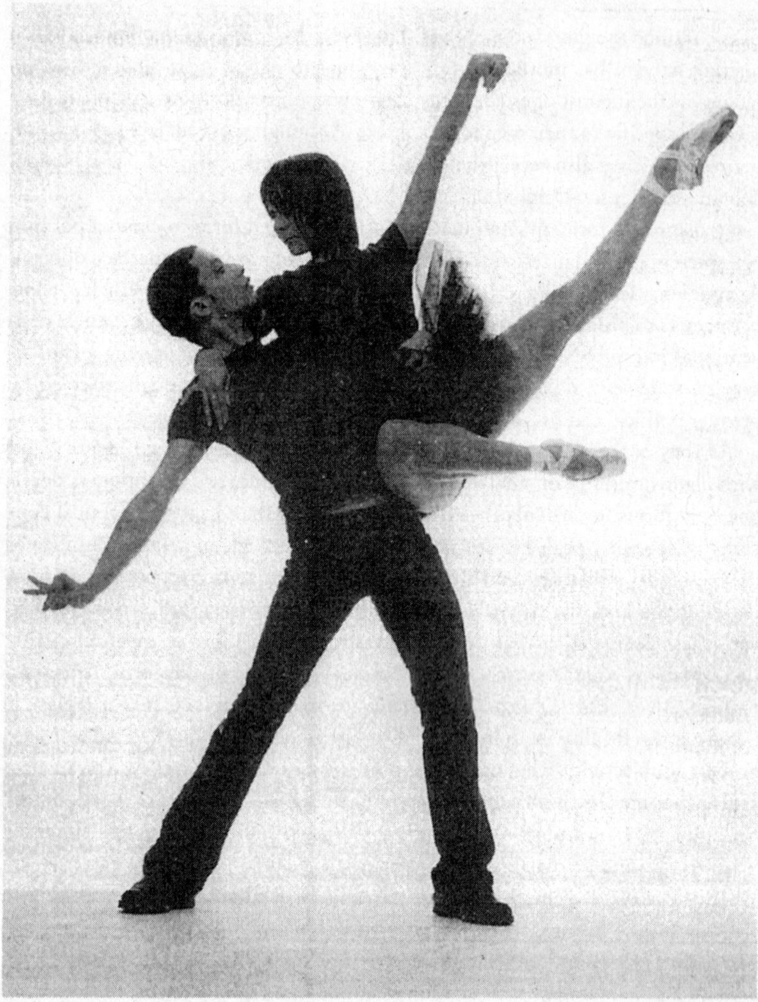

Figure 21: Mavin Khoo and Sheena Chundee. Photograph by Eric Richmond.

enabled the subsequent experiments that deploy bharata natyam (personal correspondence 1999). The choreographer Mavin Khoo suggests that Rukmini Devi's study of ballet and bharata natyam represented less a linear progression from a Western to a local practice than a critical engagement with different approaches to classicism. He has used Rukmini Devi's inquiry as the inspiration for his investigation of creative intersections between bharata natyam and ballet.

In conjunction with such inquiries, I suggest that Rukmini Devi's project was a contemporary classicist one, wherein she created new work based on the tenets, but not necessarily the form, of past practices, introducing innovations to bharata natyam that neither departed from tradition nor duplicated it. This notion of classical—as constituted by overarching values but not specific forms—allowed Devi room to experiment without compromising an aesthetic that she saw as fundamental to an Indian heritage. This reactivation and redefinition of the past lent a critical edge to Devi's project that is as useful today as it was in the mid-twentieth century. By extracting the theoretical principles from Rukmini Devi's project in the same way she extracted concepts from past practice, today's performers and viewers can promote a critical classicism that continually reevaluates itself.

The role of E. Krishna Iyer, as Sharada Ramanathan and David Gere propose, has received less attention in accounts of the revival. Nonetheless, I believe that his inquiries can also shed light on the present and future of bharata natyam. Out of his practice, both choreographic and critical, emerged the ideal of fluidity in the face of boundaries. Iyer performed this most directly in relationship to gender, by dressing and dancing as a devadasi. In the late twentieth century, bharata natyam included men but remained largely a female form. Even now, when critics and viewers attend to and celebrate the role of the male dancer, bharata natyam still appears feminized. Indeed, one of the critiques leveled at bharata natyam is that its present form demands a coquettish femininity. Iyer's practice opens not just the option of men dancing but, perhaps more important, the possibility that bharata natyam can be used to subvert gender expectations instead of reinforcing them.

The idea of variable affiliations also appears in Iyer's discussions of national and regional histories for bharata natyam. Bharata natyam, although represented through contrasting national, regional, and linguistic affiliations, remains, in critical and popular perception, linked to specific national, ethnic, and geographical identities. Iyer's performance practice and writing suggest that the dance form can negotiate multiple allegiances at once, a concept useful both to dancers who contend with kinds of difference specific to South Asia and to diasporic, transnational performers.

The present-day form can take a number of strategies from Balasaraswati as well. First, Balasaraswati, like Ram Gopal and Uday Shankar, performed internationally but did not remain on the ethnic-dance sidelines of the global dance sphere. Instead, she moved resolutely within the mainstream of a transnational dance milieu. Her performance practice challenges the international marginalization of Indian dance that carries forward today. Just as Shankar and Gopal engaged with ballet, Balasaraswati traveled in the world of modern dance. Her involvement with modern-dance venues and training institutions raises the possibility of bharata natyam's integrating with contemporary dance rather than appearing as its other. Balasaraswati's connection to modern dance prefigures the decision made by Akademi in the 1970s to align South Asian techniques with the

British independent dance sector. Performers such as Balsaraswati, Gopal, and Shankar offer the possibility that dancers can resist the exoticization of bharata natyam and other Indian dance forms.

Balasaraswati also looked to the past of bharata natyam in order to critique the present. Although she referred primarily to class and gender concerns and to the events of the revival, I suggest that the memory of bharata natyam's history can operate as an analytical device to help dancers, dance critics, and viewers investigate social and political concerns. Choreographers and dancers continually reexamine bharata natyam's complex legacy in performance, but viewers sometimes still see bharata natyam as traditional and therefore as uniform. This can produce a notion of Indianness defined as high-class, hegemonic, restrictively feminine, and susceptible to both exoticization and fundamentalism. Representations of bharata natyam that disavow its marginal past run the risk of aligning the form, on the one hand, with western Orientalist images of "ancient Eastern traditions" and, on the other, with religious-fundamentalist notions of "pure Hinduism." The nondominant narratives that Balasaraswati emphasized, such as eroticism, sarcasm, and the role of marginal women, not only offers a critique of the revival but also provides a model for drawing out other counter-hegemonic perspectives in choreography and performance.

Bharata natyam dancers, choreographers, and writers can rethink these and other strategies so that they query the practices of the present in the dance sphere and beyond. Through such approaches, as well as through ones deployed by present-day practitioners that I have not addressed here, bharata natyam can reflect on its global status in a critical, dynamic, and reflexive way. These kinds of experiments—which dancers have already begun—will continue to interrogate the conventional codes of spectatorship and of viewer expectation so that bharata natyam can truly be at home in the world.

Appendix A: Notes on Terminologies and Transcriptions

In this text, I use the most commonplace, rather than the most technically accurate, transcriptions of Tamil, Telugu, and Sanskrit words, relying on conventional Indian English transcriptions rather than scholarly transliterations. I therefore refer to the canonical Tamil poetry as Sangam, not Cankam, the epic as the *Silappadikaram*, not *Cilappatikaram*, and so on. I have made this decision because this text is not primarily a literary inquiry, nor is it located only in South Asian studies. I hope the conventional transcriptions may allow greater ease of reading for non-Tamil-speaking and nonspecialist readers.

The city of Madras was officially renamed Chennai in 1996, a shift that returned the metropolis to its Tamil name. A substantial portion of this text focuses on the refiguration of Madras in the twentieth century. To reflect this transition from English to Tamil nomenclature as a shift from colonialism to postcoloniality, I refer to the city as Madras in the revival period and as Chennai in the late twentieth century.

For cities where the change is one of more precise transliteration, I have used the postcolonial spelling throughout the text. For instance, colonials identified the southern Indian city of Thanjavur as Tanjore. I have used the transliterated Tamil name, rather than the colonial one, regardless of the time period discussed. I retain the colonial spelling in quotes and in individuals' names, such as Tanjore Balasaraswati.

In capitulation to Western conventions of formal naming, I refer to individuals cited here by their second name. I recognize that this makes for an imperfect fit with Indian, and especially Tamil, naming protocol. The idea of the surname is foreign to Tamil nomenclature, which traditionally adheres to the pattern of ancestral home, a parent's name, and given name or region of origin and given name. The first two names are usually abbreviated as initials, as in D. K. Pattammal or T. Balasaraswati. In most cases, the child carries the father's given name as their second name. Devadasis and Isai Vellala men from devadasi homes take their mother's name as their ancestral name or are simply referred to by place of origin. Under colonialism, British officials encouraged the Indian populace to adopt a European nomenclature, so some men used a caste suffix as their surname (for example, Kandappa Pillai). Others continued to use the Tamil format, such as V. Raghavan, for whom "Raghavan" is both a given name and a functional "surname." Women who follow this latter pattern generally use their given name as a first name and their father or husband's name as a last name (Padma Subrahmanyam and Nandini Ramani are examples of each, respectively).

In order to refer to performers, scholars, and critics in the same manner throughout this text, I refer to everyone by second name. Therefore, I identify some men (for instance, Raghavan or Dhananjayan) by their given name, while others (such as E. Krishna Iyer) remain identified by caste appellations (Iyer). Likewise, some women, especially devadasis and the older generation of women (T. Balasaraswati, S. Sarada, K. J. Sarasa) are referred to by given names, some (Rukmini Devi) are referred to by part of their given names (Devi), while others (Lakshmi Viswanathan) are identified by paternal names (Viswanathan). Although I acknowledge the disjuncture between naming conventions, I have yielded to this European/American protocol so that my method of identification remains consistent throughout the text. More important, I want to avoid a situation in which I identify dancers by first names and scholars by last names, because I believe that this practice runs the risk of implying that scholarship is a more serious pursuit than performance and choreography.

Appendix B: Devadasis and the Anti-Nautch Movement

Prior to the advent of colonialism, women served in a number of posts in temples and courts as dancers, singers, and ritual practitioners. In addition, several communities had family structures that diverged from mainstream, high-caste models of monogamous domesticity (Nair 1994; Srinivasan 1985). Each of these communities placed different demands on women, casting them in various roles and requiring them to adhere to sexual and domestic mores that were particular to their specific group. Likewise, the status of women varied among these communities.

Colonialists not only condemned devadasi lifestyle and performance, they also conflated a range of ritual, sexual, and domestic conventions into a singular category of the "dancing girl" (Meduri 1996). In so doing, they effaced the diversity of sexual and domestic mores of these groups. The generic term devadasi, meaning servant of god, covers a range of positions in which women provided ritual and artistic services in temples and for royal patrons. Leslie Orr (2000) proposes the use of the term "temple women" as a more accurate one than devadasi, nautch girl, dancing girl, and so on; this forms part of her argument for greater specificity in historical studies of temple dedication and the role of women therein.

In southern India, however, the term devadasi is generally appropriate in that the Tamil term for temple women was *devaradiyal*, or "at the feet of [the] god" (Srinivasan 1985: 1869). These women were dedicated to lifelong service in Hindu temples and courts. Unlike North Indian professional women musicians, such as *taiwaifs* and *baijis*, courtesan-performers in southern India remained tied primarily to temple or court ritual practices. The right to the devadasi position was hereditary and transmitted from mother to daughter but was subject to the approval of the king and temple priests. Alternatively, parents could offer daughters as potentially dedicated women; these girls were, in turn, adopted by devadasis (Kersenboom-Story 1988; Srinivasan 1985).

This text offers a brief overview of the devadasi system as it laid the ground for the bharata natyam revival. Other studies provide greater detail on the devadasi system and its historical and cultural specificities. Frederique Appfel Marglin's (1985) study is an ethnographic project based on fieldwork with the remaining devadasi of Puri, Orissa. Amrit Srinivasan (1985) combines an ethnography of the practices of the devadasis of Tamil Nadu with an analysis of the political implications of Rukmini Devi's revision of bharata natyam. Saskia Kersenboom-Story has intertwined anthropological research on remaining devadasi communities (1988) with a historical examination of the devadasi system in southern India (1987). Leslie Orr (2000) focuses on references to these women in the Chola period in South India. Aloka Parasher (1992) analyzes the temple dedication system through economic and historical perspectives. Kay Kirkpatrick Jordan (1989) conducts a study on the recent history of the devadasis in a variety of Indian regions through the changes in their legal status under colonial law. Davesh Soneji and Hari Krishnan are currently conducting research on the ritual and performance practices of the devadasis of Andhra Pradesh (see Soneji 2004).

A number of studies have approached devadasi and courtesan communities from a feminist standpoint, locating in these groups precolonial models for female autonomy (Oldenburg 1991; Srinivasan 1987). Some, while acknowledging that devadasis were dependent upon male patrons, kings, and temple officials, have emphasized the women's relative freedoms (Nair 1994) and have charted the reification, rather than eradication, of patriarchal oppression in the attempts to abolish the dedication of women to Hindu temples (Datar 1992). Others draw out the exploitation of devadasis either in the economic practices that offered them financial security—but only if they remained bound to temple service (Anandhi 1991)—or in their continued association with sexuality and/or eroticism (Post 1989).

Appendix C: Revival-Era Dancers at the Music Academy

The Madras Music Academy initially offered performances by devadasi dancers. These included the Kalyani daughters (1931, 1933), Balasaraswati (1933, 1934, 1939), Mylapore Gowri Ammal (1932), Varalakshmi (1933, 1934, 1936) and Saranayaki (1933), Bhanumati (1934, 1936, 1940), Sabharanijitham (1935, 1936), Nagaratnam (1935), and Muthuratnambal (1937). Brahman adolescents entered the academy's stage with Balachandra in 1938, followed by Kalanidhi Ganapathi (now Narayanan) and Lakshmi Sastri (now Shankar) in 1939.

Gaston lists P. K. Jivaratnam and not the Kalyani daughters as dancing in 1931 (1990: 136).

Of the devadasi performers, only Balasaraswati and Myalpore Gowri Ammal retained visibility in the performance field. Little information is currently available on Balachandra (Arudra 1986–87b: 21). Kalanidhi Narayanan reported that she was the first female Brahman to take up bharata natyam, although she did not give a date for her first public performance (personal correspondence 1999). Arudra deduces that Kalanidhi gave her first performance in 1936, based on her recollection of performing at the Dakshin Bharat Hindi Prachar Sabha during the time of Mohandas Gandhi's visit to the society (Arudra 1986–87b: 28). She is now a leading bharata natyam teacher and is renowned for her traditional rendition of abhinaya and her adherence to srigara bhakti idioms. Lakshmi Shastri has pursued a career in Hindustani (North Indian classical) music (27).

For more information on the dancers of the 1930s, see Arudra (1986–87b) and Gaston (1990).

Appendix D: Timeline of Tamil Parties and Movements

This section delineates the different projects within Tamil devotion as identified by Sumathi Ramaswamy (1997) and several major events in the development of Indian nationalism in southern India as used in this text, especially chapter 2.

1880s: Neo-Shaivism

1880s–1905: Moderate neo-Shaivism; key figure, J. M. Nallaswami Pillai (1864–1920)

1880s–1920s: "Discovery" and publication of Sangam poems sparks recognition of Tamil as a classical language. Consolidation of Tamil classicist discourses.

1882–83: Theosophical Society establishes headquarters in Adayar, Madras.

1890s: First appearance of Indianist Tamil devotion; key figure, Subramania Bharati (1882–1921)

1900s: Rise of Indian National Congress

1906: Polarization of Sanskrit and Tamil. Debates in Madras University over the compulsory study of Sanskrit and the "elimination of 'vernaculars'" (Ramaswamy 1997: 30)

1913: Theosophical Society enters politics (Ramaswamy 1997: 28)

1915: "Besant-led factions of the Congress" demand Home Rule (Ramaswamy 1997: 30)

1916–17: Founding of the Justice Party, consolidated around non-Brahman interests

1917: British promise to allow self-government in phases

1917–18: Annie Besant serves as president of the Indian National Congress Party (Allen 1997: 71)

1920s: Radical neo-Shaivism; key figure, Maraimalai Adigal (1876–1950)

1920s: Contestatory classicism

1926: Emergence of Dravidianism; founding of Self-Respect League; key figure, E. V. Ramasami (1879–1973)

1937–38: Madras government attempts to introduce compulsory Hindi study (Ramaswamy 1997: 46)

1944: Dravidar Kalakam (DK) established

1947: Indian independence

1949: Dravidar Munnetra Kalakam (DMK) founded by Annadurai

1950s–1960s: State Hindi policy

1960s: Antagonism between Hindi and Tamil; National Language Debates

1967: Defeat of Congress in Tamil Nadu by Dravidianist parties

1970s: Dravidianist parties soften position on India

Appendix E: Tamil Parties and Movements

This section provides short definitions and information on the different Tamil devotionalist movements as identified by Sumathi Ramaswamy and as used in chapter 2.

Dravidianism: A social reform and, initially, separatist political movement that emphasized the discrete ethnic, linguistic, and "racial" identities of southern and northern Indians. Dravidianism drew support from middle-to-lower-caste, middle-to-lower-income individuals with little formal education but also, because of its support of language and literature, from Tamil scholars (Ramaswamy 1997: 65).

Dravidar Kalakam (DK): Literally, "Association of Dravidians," founded in 1944 by E. V. Ramaswami; called for a Dravidian, rather than Tamil, nation.

Dravidar Munnetra Kalakam (DMK): Literally, "Dravidian Progress Association," founded by Annadurai in 1949; urged the formation of a Tamil state.

Indianist Tamil Devotion: Maintained that Tamil language and identity should contribute to, rather than detract from, the Indian nation and its independence movement. Affiliates were generally upper-caste, middle-class, and middle-income professionals (Ramaswamy 1997: 47).

Justice Party: Non-Brahman association, founded in 1916–17.

Neo-Shaivism: A cultural and political movement that asserted the "divinity" of Tamil and formulated a monotheistic, rationalist religion based on Siva worship. Adherents included non-Brahman, educated, urban elites. Moderate neo-Shaivism argued for the "parity of Sanskrit and Tamil" (Ramaswamy 1997: 30), while radical neo-Shaivism eschewed Sanskrit and by extension treated Brahmans with suspicion so that "by the 1920s Brahmans as a community were declared enemies of Tamil and of its speakers" (ibid. 28).

Self-Respect League: Called for social reform and the consolidation of a Dravidian nation and eschewed Tamil devotion.

Tamil classicism: Focused primarily on the validity of Tamil as a great classical language. Shared ranks with neo-Shaivism and included an educated middle class (Ramaswamy 1997: 28). More ecumenical than radical neo-Shaivism, Tamil classicists included Brahmans, Christians, upper-caste non-Brahmans, and Sri Lankan Tamils.

Notes

Introduction: Performing Politics in an Age of Globalization

1. Dance scholars, including Anne-Marie Gaston (1996: 224–228), M. A. Greenstein and Ramaa Bharadvaj (1998), Magdalen Gorringe (n.d.), and Mandakranta Bose (presentation, May 2004, University of Surrey), have investigated the amateurization of the arangetram. Gaston states that revival-era practitioners distanced themselves from the term arangetram but that late-twentieth-century dancers have embraced it (1996: 314–15).

2. I date the revival from the Brahman lawyer and activist E. Krishna Iyer's first forays into the field in 1923. Arudra suggests, by contrast, that the revival began in 1933 with the Music Academy's presentation of the Kalyani daughters, Balasaraswati, and Ragini Devi (1986–87: 20). Matthew Allen (1998: 80–81) and N. Pattabhi Raman (1988: 24) refer to the child dance star Kamala, whose first performance at the Music Academy took place in 1948, as emblematic of bharata natyam's consolidated respectability, so I see this date as the point at which dance revivalists had accomplished many, but not all, of their tasks.

3. A number of scholars have discussed the international trajectories of dance careers that influenced the bharata natyam revival, including Matthew Allen (1997), Uttara Asha Coorlawala (1992, 1996), Joan Erdman (1996), and Priya Srinivasan (2003). My 2003 essay also addresses this topic.

4. Texts that investigate the political ramifications of dance include Barbara Browning (1995), Jane Desmond (1991), Susan Leigh Foster (1996a, 1996b), Amy Koritz (1997), Susan Manning (1993), Cynthia Novack (1990), and Marta Savigliano (1995).

5. The dance scholar Kapila Vatsyayan, writing in 1977, argued that the revival's vanguard reconstructed bharata natyam in the process of recontextualizing it. Other writers, including Matthew Allen (1997), Arudra (1986–87a, b, c, d), Uttara Asha Coorlawala (1996, 2005), Anne-Marie Gaston (1991, 1992, 1996), Shobana Jeyasingh (1990, 1995), Sunil Kothari (1979), Avanthi Meduri (1988, 1996, 2005a, 2005b), N. Pattabhi Raman and Anandhi Ramachandran (1984a, 1984b), Gowri Ramnarayan (1984a, b, c), and Amrit Srinivasan (1983, 1985), extended this inquiry, investigating the politics of representation that undergirded bharata natyam's move to the concert stage.

6. These include Allen (1998), Partha Chatterjee (1986, 1993), Purnima Mankekar (1999), Sumathi Ramaswamy (1997), Parama Roy (1998), and Lakshmi Subramanian (2006).

7. I draw the idea of choreography as a methodology of organizing movement from Susan Foster's theorization of the semiotics of choreography (1986) and of bodily practice as thought process (1995).

8. Introducing the volume in which Chandralekha's essay appears, Ashish Mohan Khokar aligns choreography and composition: "Choreography is . . . nothing new to Indian dance traditions. . . . Choreography has been an integral part of Indian dance all along, but called 'composition'" (2001: 4).

9. The discipline of anthropology likewise enabled dance studies to look beyond formal analysis of dance works and techniques and biographical histories. One of the first influential critiques of traditional dance scholarship came from an anthropologist (Keali'inohomoku 1983). Arjun Appadurai (1996) discusses the similarities between poststructuralist claims and the tenets of anthropology.

10. Mandakranta Bose made a similar point about individual agency in late-twentieth-century classical Indian dance forms in a 2004 presentation at the University of Surrey.

11. I rely here on Susan Foster's use of Michel de Certeau (Foster 2002). A detailed delineation of the differences between tactics and strategies is, however, beyond the scope of the present study.

12. Cynthia Novack sums up the way in which dance negotiates between individual decision-making and social inscription as follows: "This is not to say that dancers consciously plan these changes; like all participants in a culture (to paraphrase Marx), they make their own dances, but within a set of rules they do not always personally create" (1990: 141).

13. Here, as in many other situations, I am indebted to Nandini Ramani for directing me to these sources.

14. Meduri also identifies a dialectical tension between Devi and Balasaraswati (1988: 11).

15. N. Pattabhi Raman contrasts Balasaraswati and Rukmini Devi in his discussion of the "trinity" of bharata natyam (which, for him, also includes the child star Kamala, who belongs to a subsequent generation): "Balasaraswati can be said to have played the role of Vishnu since she helped to preserve and perpetuate what was best in the Sadir tradition. Rukmini Devi can be said to have played the role of Siva inasmuch as, by her own and her admirers' reckoning, her unique contribution was to destroy what was crude and vulgar in the inherited traditions of dance and replace them with sophistication and refined taste" (1988: 24).

Gowri Ramnarayan also draws a distinction between Balasaraswati and Rukmini Devi, while arguing that they not be ranked hierarchically (1984b: 24–25). Avanthi Meduri raises a similar concern, urging that the two practitioners not be comparatively evaluated (2005b: 6). I agree with both writers that it is unnecessary to determine who made the greater contribution to the field. I therefore draw out Raman's insights, maintaining that the qualitative differences between these two artists fueled the revival and established the twentieth-century bharata natyam field.

Chapter 1: Tradition and the Individual Dancer

1. Vatsyayan identifies bharata natyam as both reflecting a modern sensibility and engaging with "fragments of antiquity" (1992: 8). The U.K. choreographer and scholar Vena Ramphal comments on the continuity between bharata natyam and forms that preceded it while also challenging claims that this connection to the past renders bharata natyam ancient (personal correspondence 2001, 2003). Shobana Jeyasingh also points to the confusion of origins with form: "It is one thing to say that it has roots that go back two thousand years and quite another to say it hasn't changed over that period of time. . . . Every dance has roots. Ballet has roots which I am sure would go back two thousand years if it was historically researched" (1993: 7).

2. Joan Erdman describes the intentional use of historical sources as the production of "retronymic histories" that are "created to respond to questions asked after the fact" (1996: 301, n. 13). Amrit Srinivasan makes a point similar to Erdman's when she says that "all revivals however present a view of the past which is usually an interpretation fitting in with a changed contemporary situation" (1983: 90).

3. Devadasi dance endured through this time of censure, so that pre-revival and revival-era dance practice overlapped. Gaston quotes Milton Singer as reporting that "between 1915–1919 there were at least five hundred professional dancing teachers in Madras and many *devadasis*" (1996: 65). Indira Viswanathan Peterson (1998) and Gowri Ramnarayan (1984c) note that the performance of the *Sarabendra Bupala Kuravanji* by devadasi dancers continued at least until 1944, when Rukmini Devi witnessed a performance in Thanjavur. Saskia Kersenboom worked with temple devadasis who, in the 1980s, taught her a number of their items of repertoire (Kersenboom-Story 1988, presentation at Wesleyan University 1989). Davesh Soneji is currently conducting research with devadasi communities in Andhra Pradesh (2004).

4. The recourse to ancient canonical writings set the stage for a twentieth-century phenomenon that Srinivasan (1983) calls the "textualization of dance," in which dancers debated the validity of specific features of bharata natyam according to whether they aligned with or diverged from the tenets of aesthetic theory texts.

5. This outline of Orientalist discourse draws from Edward Said's (1979) discussion of the general features of Orientalism as well as from Partha Chatterjee (1993), Ronald Inden (1990), Lata Mani (1990), Sumathi Ramaswamy (1997), and Jenny Sharpe's (1993) discussion of Orientalist thought in India, while my application of such models to dance comes from Desmond's (1991) and Koritz's (1997) interrogation of the Orientalist approaches of the choreographers Ruth St. Denis and Maud Allen.

6. I draw the idea of an "ideology of originality" from Wolff's (1987) and Roach's (1989) discussions of ideologies of "autonomous art" and of "the aesthetic."

7. Joan Erdman argues that the Indian classical dance revivals "led to a devaluation of Indian modern dance which is only today being recognized as a legitimate and important dance direction in India and the west" (1987: 80). Kapila Vatsyayan describes the paradoxical influence of Shankar: "The very fact of his having brought to light the rich resources of the tradition meant a reestablishment of the tradition and a decrying of the eclectic approach" (in Gaston 1996: 282).

8. I have reconstructed Iyer's career based largely on Arudra (1986–87a, 1986–87d) and Gaston (1996: 84–86). E. Krishna Iyer, as David Gere and Sharada Ramanathan

(personal correspondence 2003) indicate, has been neglected in accounts of the bharata natyam revival. His work, although acknowledged in the dance and music press of South India, did not generate the volume of publications that Rukmini Devi's and Balasaraswati's careers did.

9. According to Arudra (1986–87d: 33), A. P. Natesa Iyer was renowned for teaching sadir as well as the all-male Telugu language drama form *bhagavata mela* and the solo performance-storytelling form *harikatha kalakshepam*.

10. Accounts differ as to Muttulakshmi Reddy's background. Arudra identifies Reddy as "a doctor and social leader who belonged to a devadasi family" (1986–87a: 18). Gaston cites Amrit Srinivasan as maintaining that Reddy's mother was a devadasi and her father a Brahman (1996: 80) and Narasimhan as stating that both Reddy's parents were Brahman (1996: 85). Saimata Siva Brindadevi, by contrast, remarked that Reddy, her maternal aunt (1997: 5), was the daughter of a nattuvanar who taught devadasi students (personal correspondence 1996).

11. Who initiated this renaming is the source of debate. Arudra debunks claims made by both Rukmini Devi and V. Raghavan that they put the name in circulation, identifying the Music Academy's resolution of 1933 as the first official use of the term (1986–87d: 30, 31, 35). He also maintains that the phrase predates the revival because the term *bharatam* can refer to a Brahman dance master and is a Sanskrit word for dramaturgy (1986–87c: 30). Regardless of its historical precedent, however, bharata natyam emerged as the most prevalent term for the solo female form only during the revival, with words such as sadir and dasi attam retaining currency in the nineteenth and early twentieth centuries.

12. Arudra (1986–87d: 35–36) and Gaston (1996: 85) comment on the influence that Iyer had on Devi and vice versa. Arudra (1986–87d: 35) and Ramnarayan (1984b: 19) point out that Iyer invited Devi to a 1935 concert of Meenakshisundaram Pillai's disciples and that Pillai was initially reluctant to accept Devi as a student until Iyer pressed him to do so. Arudra maintains that Iyer saw Devi, an esteemed public figure, as central to the revival (1986–87d: 35–36).

13. According to Gowri Ramnarayan, Meenakshisundaram Pillai refused to accompany this performance because she had not "completed learning the main piece" (1984b: 20). Rukmini Devi maintained in retrospect that the concert was an arangetram because "she was dedicating her dance to God" (in Gaston 1992: 155).

14. Anne-Marie Gaston argues that Balasaraswati's 1934 performance at the All India Music Concert in Benares paved the way for the acceptance of bharata natyam on a national level. Gaston also notes the involvement of the American dancer Ragini Devi at the same event as a further impetus toward validating bharata natyam (1996: 82–83).

15. Ramnarayan identifies Rukmini Devi's first entry into choreography as her revision of the abhinaya for a varnam that she had been taught but with which she felt dissatisfied. Rukmini Devi also reworked *Hindolam Tillana*, a conventional dance item, relying upon her own choreography rather than that of her mentor (1984c: 26). Sarada corroborates this account, stating that Rukmini Devi choreographed new items within the margam format including varnams and padams (1985: 22). Ramnarayan (1984c: 26)

and Allen (1997: 80) also refer to Devi's introduction of *kritis*, short devotional songs conventionally used for concert music and not for dance, into dance concerts.

16. Meduri identifies this process as "indigenis[ing] and provincialis[ing] global modernity in the 1930s" (2005a: 26).

17. A review in the *Hindustan Times* (December 14, 1944) described Devi's early performances as "easy renderings of Egyptian, Hungarian, and South American dances, relieved somewhat by a thoughtful presentation of Hiawatha or a somewhat Pavlova-like reproduction of the swan dance" (in Ramnarayan 1984b: 17).

18. Gowri Ramnarayan describes this aspect of Devi's work: "She acknowledges that even in the most original of her innovations, what she had done is adapt the ancient to the new. Her unshakeable conviction is that the right foundation for true creativeness is the "eternal culture" that inheres in tradition handed down from the past" (1984c: 29).

19. Srinivasan (1983: 83) contrasts dance institutions and the gurusishya or gurukula system. Although Rukmini Devi initiated a move away from the mentor-disciple system's informal patterns of learning , Ramnarayan describes the International Academy of Arts (the early name for Kalakshetra) as providing "a gurukula atmosphere of intimate relationship" (1984b: 22) through the "medium of sympathetic contact of master and pupil" (Devi, in Ramnarayan 1984b: 22). As such, Devi became a guru herself. For instance, Ramnarayan quotes a senior Kalakshetra disciple, Sarada Hoffman, as reporting that "the student must make it a way of life to be with her and learn from her" (1984c: 33), which suggests that a student couldn't simply attend a class of a set length and expect a full inheritance of artistic knowledge, a premise that parallels that of the gurukula system.

20. I am grateful to the choreographer Hari Krishnan for pointing out this connection between uniformity in instruction and group choreography (personal correspondence 1999). At Negotiating Natyam, Chitra Sundaram and Shobana Jeyasingh both commented on the value of uniformity and precision in Kalakshetra training. See Gopal et al. 2005.

21. Peterson states that Rukmini Devi reviewed the poem at the suggestion of the Tamil scholar T. K. Chidambaranada Mudaliar, choreographed the dance phrases, and commissioned the music from Krishnamachariar (1998: 61). Devi reported that she consulted Kariakkal Saradambal, a devadasi dancer who taught at Kalakshetra, to research how kuravanjis were originally performed (in Ramnarayan 1984c: 27). Here, too, Rukmini Devi maintained that she revivified historical values rather than bringing the kuravanji back into practice exactly as it had been in the past (Ramnarayan 1984c: 27–28).

22. For example, Ramnarayan quotes Devi as saying: "It is wonderful to see how the *Natyasastra* can give the opportunity for expressing new ideas. . . . The technique in this play [the Ramayana series] may appear new . . . but every movement is according to the sastra though not presented in stereotyped form" (1984c: 32). Ramnarayan corrects the misconception that Rukmini Devi developed the Kalakshetra style of bharata natyam by reconstructing movements from the *Natyasastra*: "It is clear that Rukmini Devi did not study the ancient texts with the intent of translating theory into

practice" (1984c: 30). The senior Kalakshetra disciple and Sanskritist S. Sarada refers to the Kalakshetra style as "new" while also "concurring with the descriptions contained in the ancient treatises of dance" (Sarada 1985: 21).

23. The choreographer Mavin Khoo maintains that bharata natyam and ballet share an attention to "position over process" (personal correspondence 2003).

24. Rukmini Devi separated "international" ideas from "Western" aesthetics: "It is surprising that some people . . . actually think that we [Kalakshetra] can be international only if we teach Western music, dance, etc. . . . True internationalism in the arts is the effort to study and understand all art forms everywhere." (Devi, in Ramnarayan 1984b: 23).

25. Critics also note the emphasis Rukmini Devi gave to rhythmic accuracy as it expressed her goal of revitalization: "She certainly emphasized nritta initially, perhaps because of the influence of Pavlova . . . she became convinced that only through discipline and control—through *laya* [rhythmic precision]—could the regeneration of the art be effected, its excesses sheared" (Chandrasekharan, in Ramnarayan 1984b: 24).

26. The Kalakshetra exponent Narasimhachari, for instance, expressed a view similar to Devi's, validating change through recourse to ancient origins: "Bharata natyam is two thousand years old, how could it not have changed?" (personal correspondence 1999).

27. Balasaraswati expressed this sense of the greatness of tradition through such comments as "Bharatanatyam is an art oceanic in width and depth. I have taken you a few steps on its shore" (Balasaraswati, in Scripps 1986). Likewise, she maintained that the dance required no modification because it had already reached its apex: "And the art will continue to flourish without the aid of new techniques which aim at 'purifying' it or change in dress, ornament, make-up and interpolation of new items which seek to make it more 'complete.' This is my prayer" (Balasaraswati 1984: 15).

28. Balasaraswati presented the kuravanji that Rukmini Devi rejected—the *Sarabendra Bupala Kuravanji*—the only one in continuous performance up until the 1940s (Peterson 1998: 50, 59). Matthew Allen identifies *Natanam Adinar*, a composition popular in vocal concerts that depicts Siva in his form as Nataraja, Lord of Dance, as an addition to the bharata natyam repertoire that achieved popularity in the late 1930s (1997: 80). I have seen students of Balasaraswati perform this item.

29. Balasaraswati's improvisational ability comes across in another famous incident. During the performance of a varnam, her mridangist broke his instrument. Rather than stop the concert, Balasaraswati, knowing that she required drumming only for the abstract, rhythmical portion of the piece, improvised variations of the dramatic theme for a half hour while her accompanist sent for a new drum (Raman and Ramachandran 1984b: 22).

30. Interestingly, Merce Cunningham, who rejected expressionism and psychological narratives, also expressed appreciation for Balasaraswati (in Scripps 1986: 25).

31. For her foreign students, the tension between newer and older teaching methods made itself more manifest than for local students, many of whom received both formal and informal training in addition to attending regular classes. Although Balasaraswati launched her foreign residencies with workshop classes, once she developed a group of serious international students, she returned to modified gurukula methods of

instruction wherein dancers trained by beginning with adavus and then proceeded to repertoire, so that foreign students were able to benefit from sustained study (Cowdery 1995: 52).

32. For example, Nandini Ramani states that "Bala's pragmatic approach excluded theory as a separate and independent branch of study" (1984: 39). Several of Balasaraswati's American students comment on the emphasis Balasaraswati gave to direct practice over theoretical analysis (Karen Elliott, personal correspondence 1993; Kay Poursine, personal correspondence 1990).

33. Gaston describes Balasaraswati's perspective on "reritualizing": "She [Balasaraswati] preferred to create a devotional atmosphere for what she regarded as a stage art by using artistic elements such as suggestion and gesture rather than resorting to ritual elements used as stage props" (1992: 158). A senior practitioner of the Pandanallur style, Nirmala Ramachandran, reports on this aspect of performance: "Bala never had a Nataraja on the stage. She did not believe in that sort of thing, bringing the temple to the stage" (quoted in Gaston 1991: 158). Personal correspondence with Nandini Ramani (1996) confirms that Balasaraswati insisted that her audience and students find devotion in interior experience not through external display: "Bala said it [devotion] must be in the mind."

34. Balasaraswati's comments aligned practice and theory: "A new debate has arisen these days. It has been argued that the sequence followed in the teaching of Bharatanatyam and in the concert pattern . . . does not find place in the original Bharata sastra. . . . There is also a move to replace this structure and to go back to the so-called 'original' sastra. . . . It is amazing how, not only in art but in other spiritual spheres as well, the original and foundational concepts of the sastra-s are illumined by later-day practices that seem not to belong to, or even appear at variance with, them" (Balasaraswati 1991: 12).

35. However, as I discuss in chapter 2, bharata natyam supports a Tamil, rather than an Indian or South Asian, identity among diasporic Sri Lankan Tamil communities. Its respectability is also less apparent for these groups than for Indian ones. For many Sri Lankan Tamils, bharata natyam remains stigmatized. I have never seen, for example, an adult woman perform bharata natyam publicly in Jaffna or in the Sri Lankan Tamil community in Toronto. Mature women seem to remain in the performance sphere primarily as teachers and choreographers.

36. I draw the idea of bharata natyam as a cultural symbol from Lata Pada (personal correspondence 1999) and Ann-Marie Gaston (1996: 349). I refer to the increased popularity of bharata natyam as ironic because professional performance still carries associations with courtesan dancers of the past. For instance, it was rare, until recently, for married women to continue their performing careers. Gaston discusses the perceived contradictions between a dance career and a family life, citing numerous examples where a dancer was considered a desirable bride by prospective in-laws but is asked or required to discontinue dance after marriage (1996: 71–78). Vena Ramphal sums up this distinction: "The charge is often brought against bharata natyam that it is a sort of preparation for marriage. . . . It seems to me that the reason so many good women dancers are lost to marriage is that far from being a preparation for it, the practice of dance stands precisely in opposition to wedlock. . . . It is as if the studentship of dance

is about acquiring a cultural and cultured identity but then this process trips up when it bumps into the marital identity" (2003: 33).

37. The Toronto-based dancer and choreographer Suddha Thakkar Khandwani reported that she encountered reluctance on the part of granting agencies to sponsor Indian classical dance. This hesitation, she maintained, arose from their assumption that South Asian dance was narrative, mythological, and, by definition, antithetical to innovation (personal correspondence 1999). The London-based dancer and arts administrator Bithika Chatterjee comments on a perception in public sector funding bodies of "traditional" work as static and therefore inaccessible to "mainstream" audiences. Chatterjee also notes that private organizations, usually rooted in South Asian communities, privilege "traditional repertoire and do not welcome new work" (2002: 10).

38. *Desi* literally means "of the countryside," "local," or "regional." As Peterson argues, *desi* "denotes not genuine 'folk' forms but those that have been appropriated or translated from folk milieus and included in the canon, alongside the 'non-folk'" (1998: 41). Matthew Allen (1998) presents the debate in South Asian music scholarship over these terms, outlining the argument of the musicologists P. Sambamurthy (1984) and Lewis Rowell (1992) that the distinction is historical, with marga referring to Vedic music and desi connoting "art music" of recent historical and contemporary times (Allen 1998: 24). However, Allen also notes that "marga/desi has been reinterpreted in this century, semantically moving much closer to classical/non-classical" (1998: 25).

39. Subrahmanyam argues that ancient Indian forms exhibited a "light-footed fluency, a sense of floating in the air, an unavoidable compulsion to use more space and an ardent attempt to attain victory over the pulls of the earth" (Subrahmanyam 1979: 89). This contrasts with other interpretations of Indian classical aesthetics. Kapila Vatsyayan, for example, maintains that Indian dance forms privilege time over space (1992: 14). Vatsyayan generally holds a different view from Subrahmanyam's: despite her meticulous study of Sanskrit texts, she explicitly acknowledges that practice, historically and in a contemporary moment, diverges from theory (1992: 6).

40. Bali's approach differs in this respect from that of the dancer and scholar Saskia Kersenboom. Kersenboom has studied bharata natyam with Nandini Ramani and performs margam-based concerts in the Thanjavur court tradition. In addition, she has learned temple repertoire from devadasis of the Tiruttani temple of rural Tamil Nadu. In a performance of this material in 1989, Kersenboom highlighted the differences between temple and court practices, not only in items of repertoire but also in stylistic priorities and movement vocabulary.

41. Quoted in Krishnan 1999.

42. I refer to Krishnan's position as global not simply because he is a Canadian of South Asian extraction, but because he hails from Singapore, has undergone intensive training in Chennai and Thanjavur, and now divides his time between Canada and the United States.

43. Jeyasingh responded to the panel question "Innovation or Dilution—Can Traditional Forms Be Changed without Compromising Their Integrity?" as follows: "One of the things people say about traditional art forms is that they are 'tried and tested' and that is why they work. I would like to linger over these two words because they are not static words" (1993: 7).

44. *Surface Tension* (2000) exhibits a postmodern concern with breaking down binaries between form and meaning and interrogates the assumption that form is misleading (Jeyasingh 2000).

45. Jeyasingh discussed the innovations introduced by the nineteenth-century Thanjavur Quartet: "When [the Thanjavur Quartet] made those changes, it would be interesting to know if there was a seminar held like this. They might have had to address the same issues because whenever somebody changes things there are those who do not like what is happening. . . . There may have been many people who threw up their hands in horror and said 'I think this is terrible and we are losing the integrity of the dance form. It doesn't look like the sculptures we see around in temples, I am used to a much more ritualistic use of the dance form'" (1993: 7).

46. Hayden White's (1987) critique of the relationship between history, narrative, moralizing, and the politics of state underlies my argument that the production of histories cultivates particular politics of representation. I have developed this idea further in this book through Sally Ness's discussion of choreographic expressions of invention and cultural authenticity as they produce particular politics of representation (1997).

Chapter 2: Nation and Region

1. Musicians and music scholars have debated the categorization of South Indian performance into Carnatic versus other musics. Matthew Allen (1998), for example, deconstructs the political and aesthetic investments of the classification of music into classical versus nonclassical performance. He points out that musicians and music scholars in South India frequently distinguish between pure classical and "applied" music (1998: 27), identifying concert music, but not dance music, as "classical" (43).

2. Here I use Benedict Anderson's (1991) argument that the nation is an imagined community and that political entities construct themselves on creative, discursive levels. I expand on his ideas in order to examine the ways in which regionalists also construct their allegiance through strategies of the imagination.

3. Discussions of Tamil texts on dance did not enter the discourse around bharata natyam until the late twentieth century. Examples include Subrahmanyam (1981) and Viswanathan (1984).

4. There are some important exceptions, however, to this rule of validity through classicism. Ramaswamy argues that "Indianist Tamil devotees" believed that the emphasis given to Tamil's classicism interfered with the development of the language as a governmental and institutional device (1997: 54).

5. Here, Iyer's strategy parallels that which Ramaswamy labels contestatory classicism. If compensatory classicists illustrated the parity of Tamil and Sanskrit, contestatory classicists took this idea one step further by arguing that Tamil predated Sanskrit and thus had a greater claim to classicism. Iyer's account avoids the assertion made by some contestatory classicists that the Sanskrit texts are evidence of a "theft" of authentic Indian culture from the south by the Aryan north (Ramaswamy 1997: 44). Others have taken Iyer's challenge further. T. P. K. Sundaram counters the contention that bharata natyam descends from the *Natyasastra*, positing a Tamil history for the dance form (personal correspondence 1996). The musician T. S. Ullakanathan presents a

similar argument, stating that the Tamil tradition included its own aesthetic theory treatises but these works were assumed by Brahmans and refigured as Sanskrit works (personal correspondence 1996).

6. I draw the idea that Rukmini Devi's take on bharata natyam emerged out of both reformist and revivalist discourse from Srinivasan (1985). In chapter 3 I discuss the gendered implications of this dialectic.

7. For example, in an issue of *Kalakshetra Quarterly*, a two-paragraph insert by Devi (n.d.a) appears underneath Lakshmi Viswanathan's article "Bharatanatyam: The Thanjavur Heritage" (n.d.). Viswanathan emphasizes bharata natyam's origins in Tamil regional praxis and in Tamil texts. Though Devi does not debunk Viswanathan's claim, she implicitly questions the fundamental premise that bharata natyam is a Tamil art: "Bharata Natya is the root and origin of all dance in India. Essentially all real dancing is Bharata Natya, though now only one particular school of dance is known by the name. The most ancient authority on dance is the *Natya Sastra* of Bharata. In the south there is what is known as the Tanjore School of Bharata Natyam but Kancheepuram and other cities are equally famous for the practice of the art" (Devi n.d.a: 22).

8. The Kalakshetra exponent and choreographer Narasimhachari grew up in a rural area of Andhra Pradesh. Kalakshetra's funding system allowed him to leave his village in order to pursue dance training (personal correspondence 1999).

9. Devi's invocation of Siva also echoes the attention given to this god through Tamil Shaivism. However, Devi incorporated Siva into a conventional Hindu pantheon, while the neo-Shaivites claimed him as a symbol of a rational, monotheistic, Dravidian religion (Ramaswamy 1997: 25).

10. Balasaraswati's strategy bridges those identified by Ramaswamy as "religious Tamil devotion" and "Tamil classicism" (1997: 23). Her version of divine Tamil differs from the linguistic devotion that Ramaswamy outlines. For the religious Tamil devotees whom Ramaswamy discusses, Tamil is the favored language of the gods (23), while for Balasaraswati, it is not the language *of* deities but an ideal vehicle for expressing one's devotion to them.

11. In the Jaffna region of Sri Lanka and in the Sri Lankan Tamil diaspora, Murugan contributes to Tamil identity through his martial, rather than his amorous, exploits. According to the Canadian Tamil dancer Indumathy, the elders of her local Sri Lankan Tamil community describe Prabhakaran, the leader of the separatist movement, as an incarnation of Murugan (personal correspondence 1998). Toronto's Tamil Eelam society director, Balasundaram, stated that nationalists create songs that celebrate Murugan's battles with demons and that request his help in the analogous separatist struggle (personal correspondence 1999).

12. In this sense, Balasaraswati's project aligned with the more general significance given to "application" (*prayogam*) in Tamil culture (Kersenboom 1995).

13. For instance, Mohua Mukherjee has reconstructed a dance form she calls *goudiya nritta* that, she maintains, flourished in fifth-century Bengal and died out by the seventeenth century. She developed this reconstruction based on dance treatises, iconographic sources including temple sculptures, and existing folk practices (Ghosh 1996).

14. Both the Sanskrit and the English titles appear in the program notes.

15. Lakshmi Viswanathan characterizes *Banyan Tree* as concerned with Tamil dance, of which bharata natyam is part (personal correspondence 1999). Viswanathan invokes bharata natyam not only through the progression of the narrative, but also through the dancers' stances, torso positions, and movement dynamics. For instance, the dancers hold their spines erect and their torsos largely still in a manner identical to the classical bharata natyam position. Even in leans and falls, the torso rarely curves or contracts. Likewise, the use of outwardly rotated feet (especially, although not exclusively, for women), an overall grounded position, and the relatively static, bound, and highly articulated arm and hand positions all signal the importance of bharata natyam to the movement vocabulary of the piece. Moreover, Viswanathan quotes bharata natyam phrases and repertoire in the devadasi and revival phases of this dance history.

16. I am grateful to Parama Roy for pointing out that this portrayal of commonality eclipses caste difference.

17. I describe Chapekar's position as Nehruvian not only because she invokes the leader's slogan, but also because she choreographed a dance drama version of Nehru's *The Discovery of India* (1946), which she presented at the National Centre for the Performing Arts in 1997.

18. The nationalist investments of the Tamil Eelam Society's organizers are so fundamental, however, that they describe their work as apolitical. Although their name refers to the putative separate state on the island of Sri Lanka, they take it as self-evident that this nation exists and thus do not see their reference to it as a political statement.

19. The narrative suggests that these invaders are the Moghul forces that conquered South India in the medieval period, since the latter two groups are clearly the English and the Sinhalese. In this regard, the work conflates the histories of northern Sri Lanka and southern India.

20. Tamil devotees in India, especially during the anti-Hindi campaigns, frequently deployed the theme of an abused or imprisoned Tamil Tay (Ramaswamy 1997: 20, 101–4).

Chapter 3: Women's Questions

1. Uttara Coorlawala offers a succinct critique of the status of the classical Indian dancer as simultaneously respectable and desirable: "Expensive authentic sarees and jewellery are indispensable perhaps because they announce respectability, even as they ensure the spectator's visual pleasure" (2005: 184).

2. Mrinalini Sinha, following Tanika Sarkar, points out that the idea of an inner, sovereign realm was itself a colonial invention, not only because it paralleled the Victorian ideal of separate spheres but also because it relied for its existence on the colonial designation of its opposite, a public sphere of governmental regulation and commercial transaction (1995: 141).

3. The term post-revival period refers to the bharata natyam revival rather than to the revivalist movements of the nineteenth century.

4. The euphemism "public woman" conflates prostitution, courtesanship, and temple dedication into one term for all women who practice extradomestic sexuality. The term extradomestic sexuality comes from Srinivasan (1983, 1985) and Nair (1994).

5. The dance form's status as a feminine accomplishment extends it to non-Hindu South Asians, including Christians, Muslims, and Sinhala Buddhist women in the cities of Sri Lanka. In the Sri Lankan case, bharata natyam represents respectable femininity so successfully that it circumvents the use of the same dance to militant Tamil nationalist ends. Concerns of gender and class inform Sinhala women's practice of bharata natyam. Lower-caste men originally practiced Kandyan dance, the "national" Sinhalese form, so it remains associated with marginality (Reed 2002). Although women now perform Kandyan dance, there is no Sinhala dance tradition for women.

6. The chronicler of reform movements G. A. Oddie, although sympathetic to the goals of the anti-nautch reformers, states that the devadasis' marginality made them easy targets for reform: "The success of the [anti-nautch] movement . . . was no doubt partly due to the fact that, unlike the early marriage campaigns, it did not appear to threaten anything especially basic or fundamental in the structure of Hindu society" (1979: 108). The causes ascribed to the decline of the devadasi system are numerous. As I discuss in chapter 4, Avanthi Meduri (1996) and Hari Krishnan (2004) argue that the colonial annexation of Thanjavur in 1858 furthered the collapse of the devadasi system. Kay Kirkpatrick Jordan points out that the Anglo-Indian courts gradually eroded the customary rights of devadasis in the 1860s and 1870s (1989: 100–105).

7. Nair (1994: 3158) and Srinivasan (1983, 1985) comment on reform movements as modernization strategies. Jordan's historical study also treats reform as an emblem of modernity that in turn legitimized the putative nation-state (1989: 150, 158, 160–61, 199). Datar argues that through the anti-devadasi agitations, foreign gender inequities bolstered indigenous ones, resulting less in a feminist reform than in a consolidation of patriarchal values (1992: 82, 86–87, 89–90).

8. It is not always the case, however, that the heroine of a bhakti poem relents when her lover returns to her. In the padam *Indendu*, for example, the heroine rejects Krishna's attempt to return to her after a night's absence and berates him before turning him away.

9. I rely here on Meduri's insight about the iconicization of devadasi performers as a representation of historicity and religiosity (1996: 270). Like Meduri, I want to call attention to a continued, if sublimated, public perception that the middle-class dancer walks a fine line between commendable propriety and transgression (1996: 334, 398–400). However, rather than argue that "the devadasi" was "recuperated" into a nationalist refiguring of bharata natyam, I suggest that the enduring, if increasingly marginalized, presence of actual devadasis and their repertoire threatened both this iconicization process and the domestication of bharata natyam.

10. I base this extension of Homi Bhabha's (1994) concept of colonial mimicry on Parama Roy's (1998) study of gender, class, and caste/community-based impersonations.

11. The comparison between Iyer and devadasi dancers parallels Parama Roy's argument that the "femininity" of Sarojini Naidu and Mohandas Gandhi contrasted in nationalist discourse and that Gandhi's impersonated femininity rendered him "the better woman" because he embodied "far more fully and profoundly the lineaments of an essential Indian femininity" (1998: 150).

12. As Lakshmi Subramanian points out, "While members of the devadasi com-

munity were encouraged by the Music Academy to perform in their annual concerts, they were rarely, if ever, allowed to participate in the discussions about the existing repertoire" (2004: 25).

13. Rukmini Devi qualified her position on sringara in a 1984 interview, countering the charge that she opposed the depiction of any erotic sentiment. She specified that she disagreed only with the depiction of explicit sexuality: "Perhaps my interpretation of sringara was different from the way in which most people conceived of it" (in Ramnarayan 1984a: 23). In this interview, she also acknowledged the relativity of her moral objections when she stated that "a devadasi is inured to such things from childhood. She has seen her mother and her grandmother dance to certain things. So, even if a mudra is vulgar in meaning she may not be conscious of it. But I was not brought up that way or in circumstances where vulgarity was accepted with matter-of-factness" (23).

14. I base my reconstruction of this section of Kurma Avataram on a version of the dance drama recorded in the BBC's *The World About Us* program on Kalakshetra. I have also consulted S. Sarada's (1985) libretti of works Devi choreographed.

15. This closing image evokes conventional iconographic representations of Vishnu and Lakshmi. Unlike other goddesses, Lakshmi is often depicted as much smaller than her consort and in a physically dependent position, either sitting on his knee or, in cases where she is truly diminutive, resting on another part of his body. Other goddesses, by contrast, are depicted in a comparable size to their paramours, sometimes, as in the case of Radha and Krishna, inextricably intertwined or standing side by side (Marglin 1984: 298–300).

16. Parama Roy presents a similar argument about poet Sarojini Naidu. Roy suggests that Naidu's celebration of self-effacing heroines secured, albeit partially, her position in the public sphere as a nationalist activist (1998: 137–38).

17. Although Devi did not describe herself as a choreographer, she has been identified as such in retrospect. For example, the Dhananjayans emphasize her role as choreographic author in their article "Rukmini Devi, the Choreographer" (Dhananjayan and Dhananjayan 1986). Gowri Ramnarayan also highlights Devi's position as choreographer in article entitled "Rukmini Devi: Restoration and Creation" (1984c).

18. Rukmini Devi initiated the shift of nattuvangam into middle-class, female hands in order to minimize Kalakshetra's dependence upon Isai Vellala mentors (Sarada 1985: 50). This was a transformation made of necessity that was caused by Chokkalingam Pillai's abrupt departure from Kalakshetra in 1943 (ibid.: 49). See Meduri (1996: 366–72, 386) and Allen (1997: 64–67) for further discussion of this shift. Upper-caste and middle-class women have not completely replaced Isai Vellala men as dance mentors. Men of this community still participate in the bharata natyam milieu as teachers, with upper-caste women and girls taking instruction from them. In addition, Isai Vellala women, such as Indira Rajan and K. J. Sarasa, have also taken to nattuvangam.

19. Meduri makes a similar observation when she calls this approach "experimental" (1996: 376).

20. I learned *Sámayamide Javali* in 1996 from Nandini Ramani, who learned it from Balasaraswati. Balasaraswati included this item in her own performance rep-

ertoire ("Balasaraswati's Repertoire" 1984: 73). I base my reconstruction on watching Nandini Ramani demonstrate it in class, on my own experience of dancing it, and on a performance by another dancer of this tradition, Saskia Kersenboom, in February 2004.

21. The portrayal of bhakti through adulterous liaisons appears more frequently in Telugu poems than in Tamil ones. Tamil poems tend to metaphorize bhakti through the longing of a young, inexperienced, unmarried woman, while Telugu devotional poems include representations not only of extramarital love affairs but also of prostitutes' and courtesans' relationships with their patrons. See Ramanujan, Rao, and Shulman (1994) for translations and analyses of Telugu courtesan poems. In addition, javalis portray eroticism more frankly than padams. As Matthew Allen points out, musicians and connoisseurs generally agree that the type of sringara expressed in javalis is "plainly mundane, lacking the allegorical dimension of the human longing for the divine, which most observers find embedded within padam texts" (1998: 35).

22. Dancers have critiqued bhakti idioms from a feminist perspective (Chandralekha, in Barucha 1995 and Gaston 1996). Lata Pada reports that her young female students tend to reject the sexual double standard of this model even when it is framed as a metaphor (personal correspondence 1999). Usha Srinivasan expressed a reluctance to teach her students pieces that emphasize Krishna's philandering behavior, suggesting that modern women would find Radha's forgiveness of such infidelity inconceivable (personal correspondence 1999).

23. Uma Chakravarti (1989) argues that bhakti provided alternative modes of gender relations to that of the conventional patriarchal family by portraying the lover as a close confidant, not as an authority figure. She also suggests that bhakti broke barriers of gender, caste, and class, because it valorized devotion, not ritual purity. Finally, bhakti provided, at least for female Tamil poets, the opportunity to renounce the householder's life, thereby avoiding the gender inequities of the home.

24. I draw the idea of a contrasting problematic articulated through a similar thematic from Partha Chatterjee's (1986) study of the intersections between colonial and nationalist discourse.

25. Uma Narayan (1997) gives Elizabeth Bumiller's (1990) account of her travels in India as an example of the spectacularization of Indian gender oppression. Bumiller's text, by focusing on female infanticide and dowry deaths, emphasizes the alterity of Indian sexist practices rather than focusing on those that are shared with the West, such as domestic violence, rape, and sexual harassment. As such, it constitutes a late-twentieth-century counterpart to Katherine Mayo's sensationalist colonialist tract *Mother India* (1927). As Coorlawala points out, Veena Oldenburg raised a similar critique of Bumiller in a 1984 essay (Coorlawala 2005: 188).

26. Ananya Chatterjea critiques the "hijacking of feminism by the West" and urges the development of another model for India, "where resistance has as long a history as patriarchy" (2002). While some activists of the Indian women's movement have intentionally distanced themselves from the term "feminist" because feminism has often replicated a colonialist view of "abject Indian women" (see Kishwar 1990; Roy 1998: 206 n. 43), others insist that the postcolonial discomfort with feminism emerges out

of the same gendered separation of spheres that permits hybridity for men but not for women (Roy, personal correspondence, 1998).

27. Sarabhai was imprisoned on a trumped-up charge of human trafficking after she publicly challenged the Gujarati government to explain its inaction during the anti-Muslim riots in 2002.

28. *Stree* (*Stri*) means "woman" or "lady," while *shakti* (*sakti*) has a number of divergent meanings, including "power," especially the animating power associated with women, strength, and activeness. It also signifies the feminine principle, especially on a divine level.

29. Activists have critiqued this scene and indeed the rest of the epic because of the blame-the-victim model upon which the chastity test depends: Rama implies that Sita is at fault for being abducted and that her virtue is tainted, even though her stay in another man's home occurred by force.

30. Rajeswari Sunder Rajan (1997) discusses a parallel trend in Indian literature of the 1990s in which authors celebrated "strong women" and suggested that these heroic females have no need for feminism. According to Rajan, these authors refute feminist interrogations of society by suggesting that powerful women render women's activism unnecessary. Rajan queries this assumption, maintaining that the purpose of feminism is not simply to offer opportunities for the expression of female strength, but to eradicate the inequalities that demand such fortitude in the first instance.

31. *Kanya* represents one of Madhuvanty's first forays into the composition of evening-length works. She produced the piece for the United Nations' International Year of the Girl Child (1991) and based it on a public-service publication entitled *Meena*. I saw the work performed at Madras's Bharat Kalachar venue during the 1995 music season.

32. Gayatri Spivak refers to the split between indigenous and colonial patriarchal representations of the sati as "subject-constitution (i.e., 'she wanted to die') and object-formation (i.e. 'she must be saved from dying')" (1988: 297). Julia Leslie (1992) notes a similar divide between the colonial and indigenous patriarchal discourses on widow immolation as those that construct the *suttee*, the victim, and the *sati*, the victor, respectively. Imperialist positions on sati were complex and varied. On the one hand, colonial discourse established the idea that sati is a "women's issue" which "has fed into the contemporary feminist analysis of the issue" (Rajan 1993: 55). On the other hand, British colonialists also reproduced images of the sati as martyr (Rajan 1993: 45–48) as European, especially German, romantics, idealized immolated widows as symbols of *Liebestod*, or death for the sake of love (Figueira 1994).

33. Parama Roy, paraphrasing Gayatri Spivak, offers the reminder that reverence for goddesses "does little to destabilize patriarchal notions of gender" because the goddess-venerating Hindu public "is completely capable of reconciling the worship of powerful and punishing goddesses with the most horrific forms of gender oppression" (1998: 118).

34. Rajan uses a similar strategy to Sarabhai when she points out that none of the three quintessential "good wives" of Puranic and epic literature—the "eponymous Sati" (a form of Parvati), Sita, and Savitri—actually immolates herself as a widow (1993: 56).

35. The choice of attire invokes images of widow immolation, for the sati goes to her death dressed in her bridal finery.

36. Agni is the god of fire, and sati means either "good woman/wife" or a woman who immolates herself.

37. The shot of falling bangles references widowhood: according to orthodox Hindu custom, a widow may not wear bangles or other ornaments because of her inauspicious status. A ceremonial breaking of bangles accompanies the other rituals that solemnize a woman's transition into widowhood. The use of slow motion also introduces a poignancy that suggests loss.

Chapter 4: The Production of Locality

1. *Sabha* (organization) is the word most commonly used for Madras's voluntary arts organizations and venues. As L'Armand and L'Armand point out, sabha is an abbreviation of *sangita sabha*, or musical association (1983: 413).

2. I date the end of the Maratha period from the death of the last of the royal line in 1855. This rule was largely symbolic, however, and was restricted to the city of Thanjavur itself. The British East India Company held most of the region from 1799 until the British government assumed direct rule in 1858.

3. Milton Singer's study of urbanization in Madras provides primary documentation on this transition (1958: 369–72).

4. Raghavan's commentary and publication of the text (1945) also served to further legitimize the city's status as an arts center by reinforcing its sense of continuity. Just as the *Sarvadevavilasa* foregrounded the importance of Madras by deploying tropes and devices used in earlier literary forms, so too did Raghavan's work on the text consolidate the importance of the city. This textual study, then, helped Raghavan fuse an older, continuous tradition with a modern classical one (Peterson 2001: 25).

5. However, this transference of dance and music from the Thanjavur region to Madras was by no means complete by the late nineteenth or early twentieth century. For instance, L'Armand and L'Armand comment that the greatest period of change in South Indian music occurred in the 1920s and 1930s because of the transition of musicians from court centers to Madras (1983: 434). Milton Singer's interview with Chokkalingam Pillai suggests that arangetrams continued in the temples of Pandanallur until anti-nautch legislation went into effect in 1947 (1958: 370–71).

6. Irschick points out that the political awareness of Brahman urbanites may have developed, in part, out of their involvement in the legal profession (1986: 21). This insight corresponds to Anderson's (1991) contention that elites fueled nationalist struggles because their contact with colonizers, in governmental positions, reminded them of their subordinate status in the imperial hierarchy.

7. Devadasi dancers continued to study and perform dance until upper-caste practitioners replaced them in the 1940s. See, for instance, Arudra (1986–87b), Gaston (1996), and Peterson (1998). When elite practitioners turned to the dance form in the 1920s and 1930s, nattuvanars and some devadasis acted as instructors for the new generation of dancers (Gaston 1996; Ramnarayan 1984b; Sarada 1985).

8. These American dancers include Louise Scripps, Meda Yodh, Kay Poursine, Ka-

mala Cesar, Karen Elliot, Aggie Brenneman, and Emily Mayne, among others. Balasaraswati's seniormost disciple, Priyamvada Sankar, lives, teaches, and performs in Canada.

9. The establishment of a South Indian dance and music program at Wesleyan University contributed to the popularity of Balasaraswati's dance style abroad and encouraged international discipleship. The emergence of a group of musicians trained within Balasaraswati's family, through the instructional efforts of her brothers T. Viswanathan and T. Ranganathan, also encouraged serious performers to travel to Madras. The most renowned example of this latter case is Jon Higgins, who trained with Viswanathan in Carnatic singing and achieved acclaim as a performer in India.

10. Kalakshetra exponents comment on Rukmini Devi's innovations in stagecraft. For instance, Sarada points out that "Rukmini Devi was the first to dance with proper stage lighting in the theatre. She also arranged suitable backdrops and wings. . . . She had the help of Alex Elmore, who had an excellent knowledge of theatre art, and Conrad Woldring, who was an artist" (1985: 44). The Kalakshetra-trained dancers V. N. Dhananjayan and Shanta Dhananjayan describe Rukmini Devi's attention to space, using the classical Indian emphasis on internal geometry as a foil: "None of our traditional forms of dance theatre . . . exploit space utilisation possibilities" (1986: 30–31).

11. I derive the concept "translocal" from Appadurai's discussion of "translocalities" (1996: 192). I use this term to suggest that disparities in civic affiliation and origin can be as significant as national difference.

12. The ability of the debuting dancer to represent Indianness emerges from bharata natyam's domestication as symbol of gendered tradition, as discussed in chapter 3. The arangetram confirms diasporic identity because it concretizes a young woman's ability to embody the markers of symbolic domesticity.

13. I derive this notion of an imagined dance homeland from Jeyasingh (1995), who refers to Salman Rushdie's concept of imagined homelands (1991).

14. I discuss this phenomenon in more detail in my analysis of the practice of translation in international bharata natyam performances (2003).

15. Dancers and dance scholars comment on the insufficient honoraria attached to Chennai performances. For example, Narasimhachari discussed this problem in detail, especially the difficulties it poses for ensemble choreography (personal correspondence 1999), as did Dhananjayan (1995–96). This phenomenon, in turn, emerges out of the "dance boom" that Gaston identifies as occurring in the 1970s and 1980s (1996: 119–20). Uttara Coorlawala refers to this training surplus as part of an "overvaluation of dance and traditionality" (1996). The senior dancer and teacher Kalanidhi Narayanan refers to this as "the law of supply and demand" (personal correspondence 1999), indicating that Madras simply cannot provide solo concerts for all of its dancers when the number of performers outweighs potential viewers.

16. Several dancers—at varied levels of renown and seniority—whom I interviewed (1995–96, 1999) raised the issue of dancers funding their own concerts and, sometimes, paying venues. Gaston discusses the financial demands placed on dancers in the late twentieth-century bharata natyam milieu (1996: 234), which extends to dancers making donations to venues for the opportunity to perform (1996: 349). An anonymous contributor to Sruti's letter column, "Sruti Box," also comments on this situation in

which dancers contribute to the sabha for performance opportunities (*Sruti* 79: 3). Balasaraswati criticized this practice: "Sabha-s desire not only indirect benefits from hosting the daughters of the elite, it has even reached a pass where they expect payment for doing so. Instead of being temples for Saraswati [the goddess of art and knowledge], sabha-s have become Dhanalakshmi's [the goddess of fortune's] play-field" (1991: 22).

V. N. Dhananjayan sums this situation up in clear economic terms: "When supply is more than demand, the law of diminishing return applies. Actually, the *sabhas* do not get the revenue from the gate collection. To get over this situation, corporate bodies are approached to sponsor the shows. . . . The situation of the professional dancer is pathetic. On the one hand, they are exploited by their accompanying musicians, their rehearsal and transport charges. And on the other hand, the *sabha* organisers demand a donation to present them. Since non-professionals undercut and do anything to get a chance during the season, excellent young aspirants do not get anywhere near these organizations. . . . At today's costs, unless professional dancers get Rs. 15,000 for a performance in Madras, they cannot make a living in this profession. With regard to the proper dance drama, a minimum of Rs. 35,000 makes it worth the struggle (this does not apply to the production of a new dance drama)" (1995–96: 3–4). He goes on to discuss the role of internationally-based performers in this situation: "Their [the nonresident Indians'] need to perform and get appreciation from the people of Madras is genuine, but if they try to buy performances and reviews, it is definitely going to harm local professional dancers. They certainly have money power as compared to the rupee earners" (1995–96: 4).

The dancer and critic Nandini Ramani (1998) also comments on the complex economic factors that surround NRI (nonresident Indian) performance in Chennai, referring to the "monetary strength" of such overseas performers as they affect local costs for costumes, musical accompaniment, and recording. She discusses the importance, for international dancers, of holding an arangetram in Chennai. She speaks of critics charging for reviews and venues that "prefer dancers with large sponsorships or those who accept advertising for their souvenirs [programs]" (1998: 29).

17. This is not to say that dancers perform internationally for economic reasons alone. Further incentives include the prestige associated with international performances, the ability to reach new audiences, and the opportunity to travel. Gaston states that younger generations of Isai Vellala dancers have pursued professional performance in recent years because of the possibility it opens up for international travel (1996: 129).

18. My decision to examine the global circulation of dancers and dances through an economic lens comes from Savigliano's (1995) study of tango as an economic commodity in a transnational culture market.

19. Gaston, for instance, interprets temple festivals as deurbanizing, stating that the events are "aimed at reviving artistic pursuits outside the large cities" (1996: 335). While I agree that these events can stimulate interest in classical forms in non-urban areas, I also want to emphasize that they reinforce the importance of Chennai by demonstrating the need for an established arts center. The urban arts center offers training for dancers and the promotion of their concerts, which enables the possibility of such large-scale festivals.

20. When I attended the festival in 1996, I found that although local dancers were not excluded, they did not fill the key performance slots. This impression was corroborated by the critic Devika, who, in a review of the third annual Nataraja festival, stated that "the four-day festival featured dancers mostly from Madras, while local dancers were accommodated as they came forward" (1984: 30).

21. For instance, Devika quotes Nagaswamy as saying, "The festival is definitely devotional as compared to festivals for tourists held in some temple complexes." She also reports that "the festival was planned as a devotional offering, on the lines of the Tyagaraja aradhana festival in Tiruvaiyaru" (1984: 30).

22. The arts critic P. Orr discussed the importance of keeping forms separate in a jugalbandhi when he described a solo performance by Sonal Mansingh that juxtaposed sections of bharata natyam and odissi: "In the alarippu she brought out the contrast quite vividly. In the latter [the odissi piece *Madhuram Madhuram*], the distinction was not as clear although there was no mixing up of the styles" (Orr 1988: 9). The performance of a solo jugalbandhi is unusual and occurred only because the scheduled bharata natyam dancer, Chitra Visweswaran, had canceled.

23. For instance, Orr states that "music and dance jugalbandhis are fashionable tools used today in attempts to promote national integration" (1988: 9). The Spirit of Freedom Concert that I witnessed the year following Orr's review (July 22, 1989) likewise emphasized a unity in diversity theme in that its promotional material included the phrase "for national integration." Although the jugalbandhi incorporates a unity-in-diversity aesthetic, intercultural Indian cities play a key role in the consolidation of this kind of nationalist multiculturalism.

24. I draw this description of the contemporary urban environment as a site where the global becomes localized from Shobana Jeyasingh (1993: 6; presentation, University of Surrey, Guildford, 2000).

25. I base my understanding of Canadian multiculturalism on Dusenberry (1995) as well as on my observations during fieldwork in Toronto in 1998 and 1999.

26. Arvind Kumar wrote, in a preview of the event, that "both art forms offer more than just aesthetic pleasure. Indian art and Japanese art both share the common goal of achieving spiritual transcendence, of uniting the body, mind, and spirit" (1993: C26).

27. Priya Srinivasan (2003) points out that South Asian communities rejected the Asian American identity category.

28. I base the term unlocality on Sanjoy Roy's identification of Sinha's work (1997a) as expressing "unbelonging" and "inexclusion." Even more than Pehla Safar, Sinha's *Burning Skin* (1992) portrays the impossibility of belonging for a South Asian in Euro-Canadian society. In this piece, Sinha boils a shirt in water and puts on the scalding garment, repressing any sign of pain as he performs gestures associated with English and Anglo-Canadian etiquette such as pouring tea from a teapot and drinking it with torso erect and fingers balanced.

Glossary

abhinaya: Dramatic dance; portions of choreography in which a dancer conveys thematic content through hand gestures, bodily postures, and facial expressions.

Abhinaya Darpana: A medieval Sanskrit aesthetic theory text.

adavu: Codified phrase of rhythmic footwork; constitutes the fundamental vocabulary of nritta (rhythmic dance) phrases of bharata natyam. Adavus are also used as training exercises.

alarippu: The first piece within the conventional concert order (margam). The alarippu functions as a warm-up for dancer and audience as it introduces the body positions and basic movements that constitute the bharata natyam lexicon. The alarippu is an abstract, rhythmic piece with no thematic content.

alapana: Musical introduction with no lyrics and, usually, no accompanying choreography.

arangetram: Debut performance.

bhadramahila: "Respectable lady"; a Bengali term that reflects the late-nineteenth-century nationalist paradigm of new femininity in India.

bhagavata mela natakam: An all-male Brahman theatrical form performed in rural Tamil Nadu. The dramatic text of the bhagavata mela natakam is in the Telugu language.

bhakti: Devotion; a Hindu religious movement based on the premise that religious experience should be ecstatic, emotional, and all-consuming. Bhakti relies on metaphor and role playing in order to convey the devotee's relationship to his or her god. Bhakti forms the basis of much religiously oriented dance, music, and literature of South Asia. The bhakti religious movement developed in the Tamil-speaking region in the sixth and seventh centuries CE.

bhaktar: Devotee. The bhaktar worships the god through human paradigms of unconditional love, taking the part of the mother of a child god, servant to a king, confidante with a friend, or most commonly, a young woman longing for her absent male lover.

bhava: Mood or tone; emotional expression; term used in Indian aesthetic theory to describe the performer's depiction of sentiment.

chinna mela: Literally, "small band"; a term for the solo female dance form of the Thanjavur region; synonym of sadir.

dasi attam: A term for the solo female dance form of the Thanjavur region; synonym of sadir and chinna mela.

desi: Literally, "of the countryside." The term desi has several meanings and its implications have been debated in the fields of Indian musicology and aesthetic theory. Desi can mean a representation of the folk, subject to regional variation, or contemporary classical as opposed to Vedic.

devadasi: Literally, "female servant of god"; one of a number of categories of women who served in temples and courts as ritual officiants. These women married the god of their local temple. They did not marry a human man but lived in female-headed households and were courtesans.

guru: Mentor.

gurukula: Literally, "mentor's house"; from *gurukulavatsalam*, "living in the mentor's house." The gurukula system refers to the practice of disciples living in their preceptor's home as part of a program of long-term intensive study including both formal and informal instruction.

gurusishya: Mentor to a disciple; often used in the phrase "gurusishya system" to refer to long-term immersion in dance (or music) training under one mentor.

Isai Vellala: The caste group of which the devadasi community primarily consisted and which also produced most nattuvanars (dance mentors and conductors) prior to the mid-twentieth century.

jatisvaram: The second piece within the margam format; introduces complexity in nritta (rhythmic dance). Like the alarippu, it has no thematic content.

javali: A short dramatic piece that appears toward the end of a concert, immediately preceding the tillana. Shorter and faster-paced than the padams that precede it, the javali is also lighter and more overtly erotic.

jugalbandhi: A performed dialogue between two dance or music forms.

kathak: A North-Indian classical dance form, typically performed solo.

karanas: Units of movement described in the *Natyasastra*.

kathakali: A dance drama form of Kerala in southwest India, traditionally performed only by men.

khadi: Homespun cotton; worn during the Quit India Movement in order to reduce dependence on cloth produced in British mills.

kriti: A short devotional song. Until the bharata natyam revival, kritis were only performed in music concerts, not in dance recitals.

kuchipudi: A solo classical dance form of Andhra Pradesh, in the Deccan region of southern India.

kuravanji: Eighteenth- and nineteenth-century genre of dance drama.

manipuri: A classical dance practice from Manipur in northeastern India.

marga: The counterpart to desi. Like desi, marga has a number of meanings and can refer to practices shared on a nationwide level or classical or historical Vedic artistic forms.

margam: The standard concert order for a classical solo bharata natyam performance; consists of eight genres of dance pieces performed in a specific order. The nineteenth-century musician-composers known as the Thanjavur Quartet standardized this sequence.

mudra: Stylized hand gesture; also referred to as hasta mudra. Mudras, in dramatic sections, are symbolic and have a linguistic meaning. In abstract, rhythmic sections, they do not have a literal meaning and instead operate as a choreographic ornamentation on hand and upper-body movement.

nattuvanar: The conductor of a dancer's musical ensemble.

nattuvangam: The conducting of the musicians for a dance performance. Nattuvangam is performed using solkattu (spoken rhythmic syllables) and cymbals.

Natyasastra: A Sanskrit aesthetic theory text on dramaturgy ascribed to the sage Bharata dating from about the beginning of the Christian era.

nayika: Heroine; the female protagonist of bhakti poetry.

nityasumangali: "Ever auspicious woman"; a word for a devadasi. In conventional Hindu society, a woman's auspicious status was based on her role as a wife who had borne children and whose husband was still alive. Because a devadasi was married to a god, she remained eternally auspicious.

nritta: "Pure" dance; abstract, virtuoso, rhythmic movement with no thematic content.

nritya: Dramatic dance that interprets the sahitya (lyrics) of a sung poetic text.

odissi: Classical dance form from Orissa, northeastern India, now performed primarily by women; historically danced by temple women and *gotipuas*, boy performers.

padam: A short dramatic piece without any staccato footwork. Padams explore a single dramatic moment in detail and appear toward the end of a concert. They are more nuanced, devotional, and metaphorical than their counterpart, the javalis (Allen 1998).

parampara: Oral tradition.

pushpanjali: An opening item in a bharata natyam concert. Reconstructed from temple repertoire, a pushpanjali can replace the alarippu in a present-day recital.

raga: Melodic structure.

rasa: The overall mood of a piece; emotional sentiment; the aesthetic absorption that facilitates knowledgeable spectatorship.

rasika: Connoisseur.

sabdam: A piece that juxtaposes dramatic and abstract dance. The sabdam usually expresses a straightforward, rather than metaphorized, religious devotion through narratives of praise.

sabha: Voluntary arts organization; performance venue; from *sangita sabha*, music organization.

sadir: The immediate predecessor of bharata natyam; a technically complex, primarily solo female ritual and performance form based in the literary and music traditions of Tamil Nadu.

sahitya: Lyrics of a sung poetic text.

sanchari: See *sanchari bhava*.

sanchari bhava : Elaborations on the sung poetic text of a piece that develop the mood of a piece through tropes, metaphor, and literary references. Sanchari bhavas are often improvised.

sastra: Treatise that is religious, philosophical, or theoretical in nature.

satyagraha: Nonviolent resistance as posited by Mohandas Gandhi; a key strategy of the Quit India Movement.

Silappadikaram: "The Epic of the Ankle Bracelet"; fifth-century Tamil epic and one of the earlier works of the Tamil literary canon.

sishya: Disciple.

sloka: A Sanskrit verse. Slokas, set to music and translated into gesture, often conclude bharata natyam concerts.

solkattu: Spoken rhythmic syllables.

sringara: Erotic sentiment.

sringara bhakti: Devotion through eroticism.

sumangali: Auspicious woman; a woman who has married and borne children and whose husband is still alive; associated with spiritual power and domestic stability.

tala: Rhythmic structure.

tamilparru: Devotion to the Tamil language; used here as theorized by Ramaswamy (1997).

tillana: The closing piece of a concert; functions as the counterpoint of the alarippu. Whereas the alarippu introduces the technical features of bharata natyam, the tillana, as an elaborate rhythmic dance piece, expounds upon its choreographic possibility.

varnam: A lengthy piece that elaborates on the same structure that the sabdam introduces. The varnam also usually introduces sringara (erotic sentiment) idioms into the concert. Forming part of the repertoire of religious devotionalism known as bhakti, the varnam allegorizes affection for the god through expressions of human longing. The pièce de résistance of a bharata natyam concert, a varnam runs thirty minutes or longer and includes complex rhythmic phrases that contrast with the leisurely development of dramatic themes.

Vellala: An upper-caste, non-Brahman community, traditionally landlords and agriculturalists; associated with arts patronage in the nineteenth century and earlier.

References

Allen, Matthew Harp. 1992. "The Tamil Padam: A Dance Music Genre of South India." Ph.D. diss., Wesleyan University.

———. 1997. "Rewriting the Script for South Indian Dance." *Drama Review* 41 (3): 63–100.

———. 1998. "Tales Tunes Tell: Deepening the Dialogue between 'Classical' and 'Non-Classical' in the Music of India." *Yearbook for Traditional Music* 30: 22–52.

Anandhi, S. 1991. "Representing Devadasis: 'Dasigal Mosavali' as a Radical Text." *Economic and Political Weekly* 26 (11–12): 739–46.

Ananya. 1996. "Training in Indian Classical Dance: A Case Study." *Asian Theatre Journal* 13 (10): 68–91.

Anderson, Benedict. 1991. *Imagined Communities: Reflections on the Origin and Spread of Nationalism.* New York: Routledge.

Appadurai, Arjun. 1996. *Modernity at Large: Cultural Dimensions of Globalization.* Minneapolis: University of Minnesota Press.

"The Art of Indian Dancing: Interpretation of the Meaning of Life." 1933 (October 26). *The Times of India* (Reprint). Bombay.

"Art Revival in India: A Poineer [*sic*] Returns." 1949 (September 25). *Deccan Herald.* Unpaginated. New York Public Library Clippings Files.

Arudra. 1986–87a. "The Transfiguration of a Traditional Dance: The Academy and the Dance; Events of the First Decade." *Sruti* 27–28: 17–21.

———. 1986–87b. "Dancers of the First Decade." *Sruti* 27–28: 23–28.

———. 1986–87c. "The Renaming of an Old Dance: A Whodunit Tale of Mystery." *Sruti* 27–28: 30–31.

———. 1986–87d. "E. Krishna Iyer (1897–1968): Saviour of a Dance in Distress." *Sruti* 27–28: 32–36.

Bakht, Natasha. 1997. "Part II: Rewriting the Culture." *Dance Theatre Journal* 13 (4): 8–9.

"Balasaraswati's Repertoire." 1984. *Sangeet Natak* 72–73: 69–75.

Balasaraswati, T. 1975. "Bharata Natyam." Trans. S. Guhan. Presidential address at the 33rd Annual Conference of the Tamil Isai Sangam, Madras, December 21.

———. 1984. "Bala on Bharata Natyam." *Sruti* 5: 11–15.

———. 1988. "The Art of Bharatanatyam: Reflections of Balasaraswati." *Sruti* 50: 37–40.

———. 1991. *Bala on Bharatanatyam.* Trans. S. Guhan. Madras: Sruti Foundation.

Bannerjee, Sumanta. 1990. "Marginalization of Women's Popular Culture in Nineteenth Century Bengal." In *Recasting Women: Essays in Indian Colonial History*, ed. Kumkum Sangari and Sudesh Vaid. New Brunswick, N.J.: Rutgers University Press.

Barucha, Rustom. 1995. *Chandralekha: Woman, Dance, Resistance*. New Delhi: Indus.

BBC Television. N.d. "The World About Us: Kalakshetra." Broadcast on the Kalakshetra School.

Bhabha, Homi. 1994. "Of Mimicry and Man: The Ambivalence of Colonial Discourse." In *The Location of Culture*. Routledge: London and New York.

Bharatam Samanvayam. 1999. Program notes.

Bhattacharjee, Anannya. 1992. "The Habit of Ex-Nomination: Nation, Woman, and the Indian Immigrant Bourgeousie." *Public Culture* 5 (1): 19–44.

Blacking, John. 1981. "Making Artistic Popular Music: The Goal of True Folk." *Popular Music* 1: 9–14.

Bose, Sumantra. 1994. *States, Nations, and Sovereignty: Sri Lanka and the Tamil Eelam Movement*. New Delhi and Thousand Oaks, Calif.: Sage.

Brindadevi, Saimata Siva. 1997. "Devadasi Dancers" [letter to the editor]. *Sruti* 149: 5–6.

Brown, Robert. 1986. "Homage to Bala." In *Balasaraswati: A Tribute to the Artist and her Art*, ed. Louise Elcaness Scripps. Balasaraswati School of Music and Dance.

Browning, Barbara. 1995. *Samba: Resistance in Motion*. Bloomington: Indiana University Press.

Bumiller, Elisabeth. 1990. *May You Be the Mother of a Hundred Sons: A Journey among the Women of India*. New York: Random House.

Certeau, Michel de. 1988. *The Practice of Everyday Life*. Trans. Steven Rendall. Berkeley: University of California Press.

Chakravarti, Uma. 1989. "The World of the Bhaktin in South Indian Traditions: The Body and Beyond." *Manushi* 50–52: 18–29.

———. 1990. "Whatever Happened to the Vedic *Dasi*? Orientalism, Nationalism, and a Script for the Past." In *Recasting Women: Essays in Indian Colonial History*, ed. Kumkum Sangari and Sudesh Vaid. New Brunswick, N.J.: Rutgers University Press.

Chandralekha. 2001. "Choreography in Context." In *Attendance: The Dance Annual of India*, ed. Ashish Mohan Khokar. Bangalore: Ekah-Pathways.

Chatterjea, Ananya. 2002. "Dancing Violence through Interrupted Classicism: A Wife's Letter." Conference presentation, Dance in South Asia: New Approaches, Politics and Aesthetics. Swarthmore College, Pa., March 3.

———. 2004a. *Butting Out: Reading Resistive Choreographies through Works by Jawole Willa Jo Zollar and Chandralekha*. Middletown, Conn.: Wesleyan University Press.

———. 2004b. "Contestations: Constructing a Historical Narrative for Odissi." In *Rethinking Dance History: A Reader*, ed. Alexandra Carter. London and New York: Routledge.

Chatterjee, Bithika. 2002. "The Spin Factor." *Pulse* 3 (Autumn): 9–10.

Chatterjee, Partha. 1986. *Nationalist Thought and the Colonial World: A Derivative Discourse.* Minneapolis: University of Minnesota Press.

———. 1993. "The Nation and Its Women." In *The Nation and Its Fragments: Colonial and Postcolonial Histories.* Princeton, N.J.: Princeton University Press.

Coorlawala, Uttara Asha. 1992. "Ruth St. Denis and India's Dance Renaissance." *Dance Chronicle* 15 (2): 123–52.

———. 1993. "The Classical Traditions of Odissi and Manipuri." *Dance Chronicle* 16 (3): 276.

———. 1996. "The Birth of Bharatanatyam and the Sanskritized Body." Paper presented at the annual CORD Conference, Greensboro, NC, November.

———. 2005. "The Birth of Bharatanatyam and the Sanskritized Body." In *Rukmini Devi Arundale: A Visionary Architect of Indian Culture and the Performing Arts,* ed. Avanthi Meduri. Delhi: Motilal Barnarsidass.

Cowdery, James R. 1995. "The American Students of Balasaraswati." *UCLA Journal of Dance Ethnology* 19: 50–57.

"The Dance in Indian Sagas." 1938. *Civil and Military Gazette,* February 17. Unpaginated.

Datar, Chhaya. 1992. "Reform or New Form of Patriarchy? Devadasis in the Border Region of Maharashtra and Karnataka." *Indian Journal of Social Work* 53 (1): 81–91.

Desmond, Jane. 1991. "Dancing Out the Difference: Cultural Imperialism and Ruth St. Denis's 'Radha' of 1906." *Signs: Journal of Women in Culture and Society* 17 (1): 28–49.

Devi, Ragini. N.d. "The Survival of Traditional Hindu Dances." 67–68. New York Public Library Clippings File

Devi, Rukmini. N.d.a. Untitled entry. *Kalakshetra Quarterly* 9 (3): 22.

———. N.d.b. "Bharata Natya Sastra in Practice." *Kalakshetra Quarterly* 2 (3): 20–26.

Devika, V. R. 1984. "Natyanjali at Chidambaram." *Sruti* 9: 30–31.

Dhananjayan, V. N. 1995–96. Interview. In *Dignity Dialogue,* special supplement, *The Music and Dance Festival Season,* December–January, 3–5.

Dhananjayan, V. N., and Shanta Dhananjayan. 1986. "Rukmini Devi the Choreographer." *Kalakshetra Quarterly* 8 (3–4): 30–34.

Dusenberry, Verne. 1995. "A Sikh Diaspora? Contested Identities and Constructed Realities." In *Nation and Migration: The Politics of Space in the South Asian Diaspora,* ed. Peter van der Veer. Philadelphia: University of Pennsylvania Press.

Erdman, Joan L. 1987. "Performance as Translation: Uday Shankar in the West." *TDR: The Drama Review* 31 (1): 64–88.

———. 1996. "Dance Discourses: Rethinking the History of the 'Oriental Dance.'" In *Moving Words: Re-Writing Dance,* ed. Gay Morris. London and New York: Routledge.

Figueira, Dorothy M. 1994. "Die Flambierte Frau: Sati in European Culture." In *Sati, the Blessing and the Curse: The Burning of Wives in India,* ed. John Stratton Hawley. New York: Oxford University Press.

Foster, Susan Leigh. 1986. *Reading Dancing: Bodies and Subjects in Contemporary American Dance.* Berkeley and Los Angeles: University of California Press.

———. 1995. "Choreographing History." In *Choreographing History*, ed. Susan Foster. Bloomington: Indiana University Press.
———. 1996a. "The Ballerina's Phallic Pointe." In *Corporealities: Dancing Knowledge, Culture, and Power.* London and New York: Routledge.
———. 1996b. *Choreography and Narrative: Ballet's Staging of Story and Desire.* Bloomington: Indiana University Press.
———. 2002. *Dances that Describe Themselves: The Improvised Choreography of Richard Bull.* Middletown, Conn.: Wesleyan University Press.
Foucault, Michel. 1979. *Discipline and Punish: The Birth of the Prison.* Trans. Alan Sheridan. New York: Vintage Books.
Franko, Mark. 1989. "Repeatability, Reconstruction and Beyond." *Theatre Journal* 41 (1): 56–73.
Gaston, Anne-Marie. 1990. "Bharata Natyam: Performances at the Madras Music Academy, 1931–88." *Journal of the Madras Music Academy* 61: 116–45.
———. 1991. "Development of the Repertoire in Modern Bharata Natyam." *Journal of the Madras Music Academy* 62: 95–134.
———. 1992. "Dance and the Hindu Woman: Bharata Natyam Re-ritualized." In *Roles and Rituals for Hindu Women*, ed. Julia Leslie. Delhi: Motilal Barnarsidass.
———. 1996. *Bharata Natyam: from Temple to Theatre.* New Delhi: Manohar.
Ghosh, Goutam. 1996. "Bengal Had its Dance Form Too." *The Hindu.* March 17: X.
Gopal, Pushkala, Shobana Jeyasingh, Prashanth Nayak, and Chitra Sundaram. 2005. "What Makes Bharata Natyam Aesthetic?" Panel discussion, Negotiating Natyam symposium, Linbury Theatre, Royal Opera House, London, October 9.
Gorringe, Magdalen. N.d. "Arangetrams and Manufacturing Identity: the Changing Role of a Bharata Natyam Dancer's Solo Debut in the Context of the Diaspora." Unpublished manuscript.
Greenstein, M. A., and Ramaa Bharadvaj. 1998. "Bharata Natyam: Translation, Spectacle and the Degeneration of Arangetram in Southern California Life." *Proceedings, Society of Dance History Scholars, Twenty-first Annual Conference.* Riverside: University of California, Society of Dance History Scholars.
Hawley, John Stratton. 1994. Introduction to *Sati: The Blessing and the Curse*, ed. John Stratton Hawley. New York: Oxford University Press.
Inden, Ronald. 1990. "Hinduism: The Mind of India." In *Imagining India.* London: Hurst.
Irschick, Eugene. 1986. *Tamil Revivalism in the 1930s.* Madras: Cre-A.
Iyer, E. Krishna. 1957. *Bharata Natya and Other Dances of Tamil Nad.* Baroda: M.S. University of Baroda Press.
Jeyasingh, Shobana. 1990. "Getting Off the Orient Express." *Dance Theatre Journal* 8 (2): 34–37.
———. 1993. "Traditions on the Move." Transcript of presentation, open forum, Academy of Indian Dance. 6–9. Appendix comp. and prod. Tina Cockett.
———. 1995. "Imaginary Homelands: Creating a New Dance Language." In *Border Tensions.* Guildford: Department of Dance Studies, University of Surrey.
———. 2000. Program notes, *Surface Tension* and *Palimpsest.*

Jordan, Kay Kirkpatrick. 1989. "From Sacred Servant to Profane Prostitute: A Study of the Changing Legal Status of the Devadasi, 1857–1947." Ph.D. diss., University of Iowa.

Keali'inohomoku, Joann. 1983. "An Anthropologist Looks at Ballet as Ethnic Dance." In *What Is Dance? Readings in Theory and Criticism*, ed. Roger Copeland and Marshall Cohen. New York: Oxford University Press.

Kersenboom, Saskia. 1995. *Word, Sound, Image: The Life of the Tamil Text.* Oxford and Washington, D.C.: Berg.

Kersenboom-Story, Saskia. 1987. *Nityasumangali: Devadasi Tradition in South India.* Delhi: Motilal Banarsidass.

———. 1988. "Tiruttani Koyil Sampradaya." *Journal of the Institute of Asian Studies* 5 (2): 47–57.

Khokar, Ashish Mohan. 2001. "Editorial: What Is Choreography?" In *Attendance: The Dance Annual of India*, ed. Ashish Mohan Khokar. Bangalore: Ekah-Pathways.

———. 2004. "Long Live the King of Dance!" *Pulse* 7: 36–38.

Kishwar, Madhu. 1990. "Why I Am Not a Feminist." *Manushi* 61: 2–8.

Koritz, Amy. 1997. "Dancing the Orient for England: Maud Allan's *The Vision of Salome*." In *Meaning in Motion: New Cultural Studies of Dance*, ed. Jane Desmond. Durham, N.C.: Duke University Press.

Kothari, Sunil, ed. 1979. *Bharata Natyam: Indian Classical Dance Art.* Bombay: Marg.

Krishnan, Hari. 1999. Program notes, *Solo Works.* April 3–4.

———. 2004. "Weaving Fragmented Pasts: History, Logic and Form in the Nineteenth-Century Dance Compositions of the Tanjavur Brothers." Presentation, Barbara Stoller Miller conference, Contesting Pasts, Performing Futures: Nationalism, Globalization and the Performing Arts in Modern South Asia. Columbia University, New York, February 20–22.

Kumar, Arvind. 1993. "Indian Taiko: Bharata Natyam and Japanese Taiko Drumming Come Face to Face." *India Currents* 6 (12): C26.

Kumar, V. S. 1989. "Bharatanatyam in Baroda: From a Century Ago to Chandrasekhar." *Sruti* 62: 21–23.

L'Armand, Kathleen, and Adrian L'Armand. 1983. "One Hundred Years of Music in Madras: A Case Study in Secondary Urbanization." *Ethnomusicology* 27 (3): 411–38.

Leslie, Julia. 1992. "Suttee or *Sati*: Victim or Victor." In *Roles and Rituals for Hindu Women*, ed. Julia Leslie. Delhi: Motilal Barnarsidass.

Mani, Lata. 1990. "Contentious Traditions: The Debate on *Sati* in Colonial India." In *Recasting Women: Essays in Indian Colonial History*, ed. Kumkum Sangari and Sudesh Vaid. New Brunswick, N.J.: Rutgers University Press.

Mankekar, Purnima. 1999. *Screening Culture, Viewing Politics: An Ethnography of Television, Womanhood, and Nation in Postcolonial India*. Durham, N.C.: Duke University Press.

Manning, Susan. 1993. *Ecstasy and the Demon: Feminism and Nationalism in the Dances of Mary Wigman*. Berkeley: University of California Press.

Marglin, Frederique Apffel. 1984. "Types of Sexual Union and Their Implicit Meanings." In *The Divine Consort: Radha and the Goddesses of India*, ed. John Stratton Hawley and Donna Marie Wulff. Boston: Beacon Press.

———. 1985. *Wives of the God-King: Rituals of the Devadasi of Puri*. Delhi and New York: Oxford University Press.

Mayo, Katherine. 1927. *Mother India*. New York: Harcourt, Brace.

Meduri, Avanthi. 1988. "Bharatha Natyam: What Are You?" *Asian Theatre Journal* 5 (1): 1–22.

———. 1996. "Nation, Woman, Representation: The Sutured History of the Devadasi and Her Dance." Ph.D. diss., New York University.

———. 2005a. "Challenging the Euro-American Read on Dance." *Pulse* 10: 26–27.

———. 2005b. *Rukmini Devi Arundale: A Visionary Architect of Indian Culture and the Performing Arts*. Delhi: Motilal Barnarsidass.

Menon, Sadanand. 1998. "The Struggle for Contemporaneity: A Modern Art Form in Search of an Audience." *India Abroad* 49 (5): 46.

La Meri. 1985. "Encounters with Dance Immortals: Balasaraswati and Ragini Devi." *Arabesque* 11 (4): 12–13, 25.

Mohanty, Chandra Talpadè. 1984. "Under Western Eyes: Feminist Scholarship and Colonial Discourse." *Boundary 2* 12 (3)–13 (1): 333–58.

Nair, Janaki. 1994. "The Devadasi, Dharma, and the State." *Economic and Political Weekly* 29 (50): 3157–67.

Narayan, Uma. 1997. *Dislocating Cultures: Identities, Traditions, and Third World Feminism*. New York: Routledge.

Ness, Sally A. 1997. "Originality in the Postcolony: Choreographing the Neoethnic Body of Philippine Dance." *Cultural Anthropology* 12 (1): 64–108.

Novack, Cynthia J. 1990. *Sharing the Dance: Contact Improvisation and American Culture*. Madison: University of Wisconsin Press.

Oddie, G. A. 1979. *Social Protest in India: British Protestant Missionaries and Social Reforms 1850–1900*. New Delhi: Manohar Books.

Oldenburg, Veena Talwar. 1991. "Lifestyle as Resistance: The Case of the Courtesans of Lucknow." In *Contesting Power: Resistance and Everyday Social Relations in South Asia*, ed. Douglas Haynes and Gyan Prakash. Berkeley and Los Angeles: University of California Press.

Orr, Leslie P. 2000. *Donors, Devotees, and Daughters of God: Temple Women in Medieval Tamil Nadu*. New York: Oxford University Press.

Orr, P. 1988. "'Spirit of Freedom' Concerts in Madras: Jugalbandhi-s Promote National Integration?" *Sruti* 45–46: 9–10.

O'Shea, Janet. 1998. "'Traditional' Indian Dance and the Making of Interpretative Communities." *Asian Theatre Journal* 15 (1): 45–63.

———. 2003. "At Home in the World? The Bharata Natyam Dancer as Transnational Interpreter." *TDR: The Drama Review* 47 (1), T177: 176–86.

Parasher, Aloka. 1992. "Temple Girls and the Land Grant Economy, 8th–13th Century A.D." In *Social and Economic History of the Early Deccan: Some Interpretations*. New Delhi: Manohar Books.

Peterson, Indira Viswanathan. 1998. "The Evolution of the Kuravanji Dance Drama in Tamil Nadu: Negotiating the 'Folk' and the 'Classical' in the Bharata Natyam Canon." *South Asia Research* 18 (1): 39–72.

———. 2001. "Mapping Madras in 1800: Urban Space, Patronage, and Power in the Sanskrit Text *Sarvadevavilasa*." Presentation for panel "From Madras to Chennai: The City That Milton Singer Never Saw," annual meeting of the Association for Asian Studies, Chicago, March 25.

Post, Jennifer. 1989. "Professional Women in Indian Music: The Death of the Courtesan Tradition." In *Women and Music in Cross-Cultural Perspective*, ed. Ellen Koskoff. Urbana: University of Illinois Press.

Raghavan, V. 1945. "Some Musicians and their Patrons About 1800 A.D. in Madras City." *Music Academy Journal* 16: 127–33.

———. 1974. "Bharata Natya." *Music Academy Journal* 45: 233–62.

Raman, N. Pattabhi. 1988. "The Trinity of Bharatanatyam: Bala, Rukmini Devi, and Kamala." *Sruti* 48: 23–24.

———. 2001. "What Is Bharata Natyam?" *Sruti* 203: 21–29.

Raman, N. Pattabhi, and Anandhi Ramachandran. 1984a. "Balasaraswati: The Whole World in Her Hands: Part 1." *Sruti* 4: 17–30.

———. 1984b. "Balasaraswati: The Whole World in Her Hands: Part 2." *Sruti* 5: 17–31.

Ramani, Nandini. 1984. "Bala: My Guru." Interview by Gowri Ramnarayan. *Sruti* 5: 35–39.

———. 1998. "Discordant Steps." *Hindu Folio*, 28–31. December 27.

Ramanujan, A. K., Velcheru Narayana Rao, and David Shulman, trans. and eds. 1994. *When God Is a Customer: Telugu Courtesan Songs*. Berkeley: University of California Press.

Ramaswamy, Sumathi. 1997. *Passions of the Tongue: Language Devotion in Tamil India, 1891–1970*. Berkeley and Los Angeles: University of California Press.

Ramnarayan, Gowri. 1984a. "Rukmini Devi: A Quest for Beauty." *Sruti* 8: 17–29.

———. 1984b. "Rukmini Devi: Dancer and Reformer." *Sruti* 9: 17–29.

———. 1984c. "Rukmini Devi: Restoration and Creation." *Sruti* 10: 26–38.

Ramphal, Vena. 2003. "Rukmini Devi Revisited." *Dance Theatre Journal* 19 (3): 31–41.

Rao, Maya. 2001. "What Is Choreography?" In *Attendance: The Dance Annual of India*, ed. Ashish Mohan Khokar. Bangalore: Ekah-Pathways.

Reed, Susan A. 2002. "Performing Respectability: The Berava, Middle-Class Nationalism, and the Classicization of Kandyan Dance in Sri Lanka." *Cultural Anthropology* 17 (2): 246–76.

Roach, Joseph. 1989. "Theatre History and the Ideology of the Aesthetic." *Theatre Journal* 41 (2): 155–68.

Roy, Parama. 1998. *Indian Traffic: Identities in Question in Colonial and Postcolonial India*. Berkeley and Los Angeles: University of California Press.

Roy, Sanjoy. 1997a. "Dirt, Noise, Traffic: Contemporary Indian Dance in the Western City; Modernity, Ethnicity, and Hybridity." In *Dance in the City*, ed. Helen Thomas. New York: St. Martin's Press.

Rubidge, Sarah. 1996. *Romance . . . with Footnotes*. London: Shobana Jeyasingh Dance Company.

Rushdie, Salman. 1991. "Imaginary Homelands." In *Imaginary Homelands: Essays and Criticism, 1981–1991*. London: Granta Books.

Sangari, Kumkum. 1987. "There Is No Such Thing as a Voluntary Sati." *The Times of India*, October 25.

———. 1989. "Introduction: Representations in History." *Journal of Arts and Ideas* 17–18: 3–7.

Said, Edward. 1979. *Orientalism*. New York: Vintage.

Sarada, S. 1985. *Kalakshetra Rukmini Devi*. Madras: Kala Mandir Trust.

———. 1996. "Advice from a Veteran." Interview by Indu. *Sruti* 136: 15–22.

Savigliano, Marta E. 1995. *Tango and the Political Economy of Passion*. Boulder, Colo.: Westview Press.

Scripps, Louise Elcaness, ed. 1986. *Balasaraswati: A Tribute to the Artist and Her Art* [pamphlet]. Balasaraswati School of Music and Dance.

Seetha, S. 1981. *Tanjore as a Seat of Music (During the 17th, 18th, and 19th Centuries)*. Madras: University of Madras Press.

Sethuraman, R. 1985. "Sucheta Chapekar's Experiment: Synthesis of Bharatanatyam and Hindustani Music." *Sruti* 20 & 20-S: 43–46.

Sharpe, Jenny. 1993. *Allegories of Empire: The Figure of Woman in the Colonial Text*. Minneapolis: University of Minnesota Press.

Singer, Milton. 1958. "The Great Tradition in a Metropolitan Center: Madras." *Journal of American Folklore* 71 (281): 349–88.

Sinha, Mrinalini. 1995. "Potent Protests: The Age of Consent Controversy, 1891." In *Colonial Masculinity: The "Manly Englishman" and the "Effeminate Bengali" in the Late Nineteenth Century*. Manchester and New York: Manchester University Press.

Soneji, Davesh. 2004. "Living History: Performing Memory: Devadasi Women in Telugu-Speaking South India." *Dance Research Journal* 36 (2): 30–49.

Spivak, Gayatri Chakravorty. 1988. "Can the Subaltern Speak?" In *Marxism and the Interpretation of Culture*, ed. Cary Nelson and Lawrence Grossberg. Urbana: University of Illinois Press.

———. 1999. "Literature." In *A Critique of Postcolonial Reason: Toward a History of a Vanishing Present*. Cambridge, Mass.: Harvard University Press.

Srinivasan, Amrit. 1983. "The Hindu Temple-Dancer: Prostitute or Nun?" *Cambridge Anthropology* 8 (1): 73–99.

———. 1985. "Reform and Revival: The Devadasi and Her Dance." *Economic and Political Weekly* 20 (44): 1869–76.

———. 1987. "Women and the Reform of Indian Tradition: Gandhian Alternative to Liberalism." *Economic and Political Weekly* 22 (51): 2225–28.

Srinivasan, Priya. 2003. "Performing Indian Dance in America: Interrogating Modernity, Tradition, and the Myth of Cultural Purity." Ph.D. diss., Northwestern University.

Subramanian, Lakshmi. 2004. "From the Tanjore Court to the Madras Academy: The Making of a Modern Classical Tradition." Keynote address at Contesting Pasts, Performing Futures: Nationalism, Globalization and the Performing Arts in Modern South Asia. Columbia University, New York.

———. 2006. *From the Tanjore Court to the Madras Music Academy: A Social History of Music in South India*. Delhi: Oxford University Press.

Subrahmanyam, Padma. 1979. *Bharata's Art, Then and Now*. Madras: Intermedia.

———. 1981. "Inscriptions in Tamilnadu Relating to Dance." *Journal of the Music Academy* 52: 122–31.

Sunder Rajan, Rajeswari. 1993. *Real and Imagined Women: Gender, Culture and Postcolonialism*. London and New York: Routledge.

———. 1997. "Contemporary Indian Fiction in English and the Crisis of Feminism." Presented at Re-Presenting Women: Women in the Literary, Performing and Visual Arts of India conference, University of California, Berkeley, April 26.

Terada, Yoshitaka. 2000. "T. N. Rajarattinam Pillai and Caste Rivalry in South Indian Classical Music." *Ethnomusicology* 44 (3): 460–90.

Vatsyayan, Kapila. 1977. *Classical Indian Dance in Literature and the Arts*. New Delhi: Sangeet Natak Akademi.

———. 1992. *Indian Classical Dance*. New Delhi: Publications Division, Ministry of Information and Broadcasting, Government of India.

Viswanathan, Lakshmi. N.d. "Bharatanatyam: The Thanjavur Heritage." *Kalakshetra Quarterly* 9 (3): 20–22.

———. 1984. *Bharatanatyam: The Tamil Heritage*. Madras: Sri Kala Chakra Trust.

Visweswaran, Kamala. 1994. *Fictions of Feminist Ethnography*. Minneapolis: University of Minnesota Press.

White, Hayden. 1987. "The Value of Narrativity in the Representation of Reality." In *The Content of the Form: Narrative Discourse and Historical Representation*. Baltimore, Md.: Johns Hopkins University Press.

Wolff, Janet. 1987. "Foreword: The Ideology of Autonomous Art." In *Music and Society: The Politics of Composition, Performance, and Reception*, ed. Richard Leppert and Susan McClary. Cambridge: Cambridge University Press.

Index